Healing Your Inner Child

A Comprehensive Guide to Healing Your Inner Child: Overcome Trauma, Embrace Self-Love, and Achieve Lasting Emotional Freedom

Dan.G

TABLE OF CONTENTS

INTRODUCTION

Every bruise we carry from childhood outlines a story begging to be heard. What unseen bruises and marks do your body and mind hold? Healing emotional wounds from childhood is a personal and challenging journey, and it's one that many embark upon feeling lost or stuck in unhealthy patterns.

Imagine a small version of yourself, perhaps sitting quietly in a corner, waiting patiently to be hugged. This little one holds the keys to your joy, creativity, and healing and is eager to be rediscovered. The inner child represents the purest part of ourselves: our innocence, spontaneity, and authentic self, often overshadowed by layers of emotional pain and defenses built up over the years. You need to reconnect with this part of yourself if you want to experience personal growth and happiness. It's about nurturing the parts of you that have been neglected and giving space for those buried emotions to surface. When you really see your inner child, you lay the foundation for progress toward emotional freedom.

Now, think about what would happen if you approach your inner child with curiosity instead of judgment. What would happen if you allowed yourself to ask questions and hear the whispers of your own stories? The answers may surprise you. It's about inviting openness and curiosity to the discussion so you let go of preconceived notions and become willing to explore uncharted territories within yourself. An inquisitive mind and an open heart create a safe space for self-discovery and healing.

The path to healing is rarely a straight line. You might encounter feelings of fear or insecurity that echo the childhood experiences you wish to leave behind. It's okay to feel this way. Discomfort, self-doubt, and a range of emotions that can be challenging to work through are part of the healing process. However, it's important to acknowledge these struggles. Understanding that these feelings are valid and shared by many others can help you move forward with self-compassion.

Consider how it might feel to acknowledge even the slightest progress in your healing journey. Each step forward is a victory to celebrate—a flicker of light guiding you through the darkness. Healing is a continual process, and recognizing every bit of progress nurtures resilience and motivation. Celebrating milestones reinforces the positive changes you're making, no matter how minor they seem. You build momentum and encourage yourself to keep moving forward, even when it's tough.

As you turn the pages ahead, remember that each exercise is a step forward. Think of this book as your toolbox, where every tool and action empowers you to reconstruct the basis of your emotional health. Healing demands active participation instead of the passive consumption of information. Actionable steps are essential because they put theory into practice and allow you to make tangible progress. Each practical exercise, reflection prompt, and strategy is designed to help you take ownership of your emotional well-being.

The good news is that healing doesn't have to be lonely. As we go on a journey of self-exploration together, envision a circle of fellow travelers around you, each sharing their stories, strengths, and vulnerabilities. A sense of community is vital because it helps us realize we are not alone in our experiences. Sharing stories and connecting with others who understand our struggles can offer comfort and encouragement. Embrace the collective aspect of healing and know that you are part of a broader group of people who want emotional freedom and growth.

This book is a companion on your healing journey. Whether you're an adult who needs guidance healing, a mental health practitioner supporting clients, or someone interested in personal development, mindfulness, and emotional well-being, this book is designed to help you by offering concrete steps to rekindle your connection with your inner child. Each chapter, exercise, and piece of advice is crafted to support you as you delve into the depths of your past, confront old wounds, and emerge with a renewed sense of self. Your inner child beckons you with the promise of joy, creativity, and wholeness, and as you proceed, you'll find that reconnecting with this part of yourself can transform your life.

Remember, the bruises of your childhood tell stories that deserve to be heard, and through this process, you'll find the strength to rewrite them with compassion and love. It's time to unlock the doors to your most profound healing and witness the remarkable transformation that awaits

1

Understanding
the Inner Child

Your inner child represents the core emotional and psychological aspects of your childhood experiences, holding both your happiest memories and deepest pains. By reconnecting with this part of yourself, you can uncover the emotions that have been buried and understand how they affect your adult life. Acknowledging your inner child allows you to confront unresolved issues from your past and opens the door to immense healing and transformation.

Where Does the Inner Child Come From?

The concept of the inner child is essential to understanding emotional healing, especially for those who have experienced trauma or neglect during their formative years. The inner child is a storage center of our earliest encounters with the world and includes both joyful and painful memories. By acknowledging the inner child, we can identify unresolved emotions that may affect our adult lives.

Historic Roots

Historically, the idea of the inner child is rooted in psychological theory. Carl Jung introduced the concept of the "divine child" archetype, reflecting an innate, universal part of the human psyche. He said that people have basic images in their unconscious minds that affect their thinking and actions (Rohde-Brown, 2023). In modern therapy, this idea has changed into what we call the inner child, and recognizing this part of ourselves helps us deal with deep emotional pain from early life experiences.

Therapists like Alice Miller and John Bradshaw made the term more common in modern psychology. They showed how unmet needs and trauma from childhood can affect adults. Miller's work emphasized the importance of facing and accepting these childhood experiences instead of hiding them to become emotionally healthy (Wedge, 2021). Bradshaw focused on the need for "reparenting," which means adults learn to care for their unmet childhood needs through kindness and support to themselves (Grist, 2020).

Introducing Therapeutic Approaches

We'll discuss various therapeutic approaches in Chapter 7, but now is a good time to introduce some of them. Therapy offers different interpretations and methods to connect with the inner child. Cognitive behavioral therapy (CBT) focuses on identifying and altering negative thought patterns that stem from childhood. CBT practitioners help clients recognize how past experiences shape their current mindset and behaviors. In contrast, psychodynamic therapy delves deeper into the unconscious mind and explores the impact of repressed memories and emotions from childhood to uncover and process these hidden feelings.

Play therapy, often used with children, also provides valuable insights for adults reconnecting with their inner child. Playful activities can evoke forgotten emotions and instill a sense of safety and creativity. Techniques like visualization and guided imagery are commonly used to help clients imagine comforting scenarios for their inner child and to encourage emotional healing.

Culture's Perspective

Cultural narratives influence our understanding of the inner child, but they vary widely across different societies and impact how we perceive our childhood experiences. For instance, in many Western cultures, there is a strong emphasis on individuality and personal achievement. As a result, emotional struggles stemming from childhood might be viewed as personal failure or inadequacy. Conversely, collectivist cultures, which prioritize communal support and interdependence, may offer more integrated and supportive frameworks to address childhood trauma.

Understanding cultural contexts is important for creating inclusivity and connecting to personal experiences.

Indigenous communities, for example, often have storytelling traditions that showcase their history and strength. The idea of historical trauma shows how shared experiences of colonization and displacement affect people's well-being and emphasizes the importance of cultural identity in building resilience against challenges.

A clear life story can help reduce negative outcomes like suicide risk (Lew et al., 2020). The idea of cultural continuity focuses on actions that reflect a community's shared history and values, which can support the mental health of individuals. Mental health professionals who include these cultural stories in therapy can develop more effective and compassionate methods to help their patients heal.

Eastern philosophies also offer valuable ideas about the inner child. The concept of karma in Hindu and Buddhist beliefs suggests that unmet desires and unresolved issues from past lives affect our current situation. This view, which is similar to Jungian ideas about the subconscious, emphasizes spiritual growth. Healing the inner child involves breaking these cycles through mindfulness, meditation, and self-care.

The Psychological Impact of Childhood Experiences

Early experiences shape our sense of self and emotions and help us understand our current struggles. Your personality is formed mainly during childhood through interactions with caregivers, family, and the community. Children who receive consistent love and support usually develop a positive self-image and healthy emotions. In contrast, those who experience neglect or criticism frequently feel inadequate, which can harm their self-esteem and emotional well-being later in life.

Different types of childhood trauma, both obvious and subtle, can significantly affect your emotional health. Obvious traumas, like physical or sexual abuse, are easier to identify but not necessarily more harmful than subtle traumas, such as emotional neglect or regular criticism. These subtler traumas can affect a child's sense of safety. For example, a child who is often told they are not good enough may grow up doubting their abilities, which can lead to anxiety and depression.

Unhealed emotional wounds from childhood can show up in adult behavior and relationships, demonstrating why taking responsibility for your healing is important. Unresolved trauma can appear in various ways, like finding it difficult to deal with your emotions, struggling to form strong relationships, or engaging in self-destructive behavior. For example, someone who dealt with abandonment as a child might find it hard to trust others and have a fear of rejection. Once you recognize these patterns, you can take steps toward healing by understanding how your past experiences relate to your current challenges.

The idea is that linking past experiences with present behavior increases self-awareness and shows how healing the inner child can positively affect adult life. This means recognizing how early experiences influence our reactions today. For instance, someone with a critical parent could be very hard on themselves as an adult, which affects their confidence. Connections between the past and present can help you tackle these deep issues, increase self-awareness, and create emotional freedom.

You need to take responsibility for your healing journey by looking at the roots of negative behaviors and actively trying to change them. It may require professional help, like therapy, to uncover and confront buried feelings using techniques like cognitive behavioral therapy to recognize and change harmful thinking patterns for healthier behavior and emotional responses. Therapists who focus on childhood trauma can provide tailored strategies to help you navigate this complex process. Techniques like dialectical behavior therapy (DBT) and eye movement desensitization and reprocessing (EMDR) can help address deep emotional wounds so that you develop healthier emotional responses.

Early experiences can also help explain why certain situations trigger intense emotional reactions. For example, a person who felt unsafe as a child may feel extreme anxiety in settings they consider potentially dangerous, even if there is no real threat. You can better manage your emotions when you identify these triggers. The long-lasting effects of unaddressed childhood experiences can lead to mental health issues like depression and anxiety. It can even cause physical health problems, such as heart disease, as the stress from trauma can harm the body over time.

To deal with these issues, it can help to create a routine for self-reflection and emotional management. Techniques like mindfulness meditation or journaling can assist you in reconnecting with your inner child, providing a safe place to heal old wounds. Creative activities, like art or music, can also be therapeutic and allow for emotional expression.

Building resilience is also crucial in addressing childhood trauma, as thinking about it can knock you down, and you have no choice but to get up again. Resilience isn't something you're born with, but it is a skill that can be developed through supportive relationships, positive experiences, and healthy coping strategies. For example, joining support groups or community activities can give you a sense of belonging and strengthen your ability to overcome challenges.

It takes time and kindness to heal your inner child. You have to treat yourself with the same care and understanding you would offer a distressed child. This could mean speaking kindly to yourself, celebrating small successes, and allowing for mistakes without harsh criticism.

How the Inner Child Shapes Adult Behavior

It's been mentioned already, but your inner child can affect your behavior today. You might even realize that certain actions aren't okay and that they stem from your childhood. Let's take a closer look at this situation:

Behavioral Patterns Emerging From Childhood

Many adults find themselves trapped in self-sabotage cycles, a behavior that often has roots in suppressed emotions from childhood. These behaviors are defense mechanisms we created to protect ourselves from pain or disappointment when we were young. For instance, a child who continually experiences rejection may develop a fear of failure and employ self-sabotage as an unconscious way to avoid getting hurt again. The fear of failure (or other feelings or behavior) has become ingrained in the brain's wiring patterns to ensure survival during childhood, but in adulthood, the brain doesn't know the difference, resulting in actions that undermine success and happiness.

Another common example is perfectionism. Someone whose inner child felt unloved unless they achieved perfect results might become an adult who sets impossibly high standards. They feel like failures when these standards aren't met, which reinforces a cycle of self-sabotage and low self-worth. To break these unhealthy cycles, it's important to recognize the emotions and memories behind these tendencies. Awareness allows us to rewrite our stories and adopt healthier habits.

Impact on Relationships

Childhood dynamics influence interpersonal relationships and may create adult attachment styles, which range from secure to various forms of insecurity, like anxious, ambivalent, or avoidant attachments. If a child experiences inconsistent care or neglect, they might develop an anxious attachment style and frequently look for validation or fear abandonment in their adult relationships. Alternatively, those who faced emotional unavailability from caregivers might adopt an avoidant attachment style, distancing themselves from others to shield against potential pain.

Attachment styles shape how we connect with others and manage conflicts. An adult with a disorganized attachment style might flip between clinginess and distant behavior, which makes stable relationships challenging. However, recognizing these patterns helps you address underlying issues and creates healthier and more fulfilling connections. Through therapy, you can learn to identify and challenge maladaptive thoughts, paving the way for more positive interactions.

Coping Mechanisms Developed in Childhood

Coping strategies forged during childhood can be lifesavers at the time but become detrimental if carried into adulthood. These mechanisms are often survival tactics that help a child work through difficult situations, but they were never meant for long-term use. A classic example is emotional detachment: A child growing up in a tumultuous environment may shut down emotions as a way to cope with chaos or abuse. However, continuing this practice into adulthood results in emotional numbness and difficulty forming intimate relationships.

Similarly, people-pleasing may come from a childhood need to keep peace or earn love from demanding caregivers. While it might have ensured safety then, it can result in burnout and resentment in adulthood as the individual constantly prioritizes others over themselves. We need to identify these coping mechanisms and replace them with healthier alternatives. Techniques like mindfulness and journaling can help uncover these ingrained habits and enable a shift toward more adaptive responses.

Revisiting Core Beliefs Established in Childhood

Core beliefs are deep-seated convictions formed during early years that influence our thought processes and self-perception. These beliefs often stem from repeated messages received in childhood. For instance, a child frequently criticized for mistakes may internalize the belief, "I am not good enough," which can haunt their adult life and manifest as chronic self-doubt and fear of taking risks.

We must address and challenge these outdated beliefs to create a healthier self-identity. An effective method is cognitive restructuring, a CBT technique where you identify negative thought patterns and systematically challenge their validity. You can gradually reframe your self-concept by questioning the evidence supporting these beliefs and considering alternative viewpoints.

For example, someone who believes, "I am unlovable because I was rejected as a child," can recognize instances of affection and acceptance in their current life. This change in perspective helps to cultivate self-compassion and a more balanced self-view. Affirmations and self-love can further reinforce positive beliefs, nurturing a stronger sense of worth and identity.

Common Signs of an Unhealed Inner Child

To heal your inner child, you must first recognize the signs that this part of you may still be wounded. These indicators can guide you toward identifying and addressing unresolved childhood issues so that you can heal and have healthier adult relationships. We're going to look at a few of these signs, how to identify them, and some beginner strategies to cope better, but these coping mechanisms will be discussed in later chapters.

Typical Emotional Reactions

Emotional overreactions, such as excessive anger or sadness, often signal unresolved pain from childhood. For instance, if you find yourself losing control over minor inconveniences or displaying intense emotional reactions to certain things, it might be a reflection of deeper wounds. These reactions are your inner child's way of expressing unaddressed emotions and unmet needs.

Spend time exploring the origins of these feelings to reveal more about your past traumas. Make notes of any situations or interactions that elicit strong emotional responses. Ask yourself why these instances provoke such intense reactions. What do they remind you of from your childhood? The identification process can help you uncover deep-seated issues and get you ready to manage overwhelming emotions.

Patterns of Anxiety and Fear

Issues related to anxiety and fear often come from unresolved childhood experiences. For example, recurring fears of abandonment or social anxiety could indicate past neglect or traumatic incidents. Recognizing these patterns enables you to address the underlying fears manifesting in your adult life. Start by acknowledging your fears by consciously recognizing and naming the fears you experience in different scenarios. Reflect on your childhood to identify any events or experiences that may have contributed to these fears; the more specific you can be, the better. Work on coping strategies to help you manage anxiety, such as deep breathing exercises, mindfulness, or grounding techniques.

Struggles With Self-Worth and Self-Compassion

Low self-worth and a lack of self-compassion are frequently linked to validation issues experienced during childhood (Ferguson, 2022). If you struggle with feeling good enough or constantly look for approval from others, it might be traced back to times when your achievements were overlooked or when you felt unappreciated as a child. Self-love and self-compassion can change how you perceive yourself and your abilities. At a minimum, regularly remind yourself of your strengths and accomplishments. It can help to develop a habit of acknowledging your efforts and successes rather than waiting for external validation; in other words, if you know you did something well, celebrate it. Activities like writing letters to your inner child also affirm love and acceptance, so you might want to include everything you wish someone had told you as a child.

Repetitive Unhealthy Relationship Dynamics

Unresolved childhood issues often cause recurring unhealthy patterns in relationships. For instance, continuously finding yourself in relationships where you feel undervalued or mistreated can indicate persistent inner child wounds. However, recognizing these cycles can motivate you to make meaningful changes that result in healthier relationships. Think about your past and current relationships and the roles you tend to assume to identify any similarities or recurring themes. Determine if any aspects of these relationships mirror dynamics from your upbringing, and learn to establish and communicate clear boundaries to protect your emotional well-being.

Examples of Indicators

To better understand these concepts, let's examine some common ways inner child wounds may appear. Addiction, whether to substances, food, or work, can be an attempt to fill a void left by unmet needs during childhood. A constant need to be in control or trust issues may suggest a lack of security during childhood. The "never enough" syndrome, where you constantly seek admiration, can link back to a childhood devoid of sufficient appreciation or validation.

Fears of abandonment often signify past experiences of being left alone or not having sufficient emotional support. You may have difficulty setting boundaries or expressing emotions, which can be traced to environments where your feelings were dismissed or shamed. Social anxiety or becoming overly competitive might reflect a need to prove your worth, stemming from a lack of recognition or encouragement during early years. These indicators shed light on past experiences and equip you with the knowledge to address them effectively. Although it's tough to revisit and process painful memories, it leads to greater emotional freedom and healthier relationships.

Importance of Reconnecting With Your Inner Child

Many adults carry wounds and unmet needs from their early years that manifest in their current relationships and behaviors. Only when they address these unresolved issues can they create healthier interactions with others and have a more joyous life. Right now, we will focus on the importance of establishing a connection with the inner child, and in later chapters, we'll discuss how to do it.

Reconnecting with our inner child allows us to revisit those vulnerable moments from our past that have shaped who we are. Imagine a child who felt ignored or unappreciated; as an adult, this person may feel inadequate or constantly want approval from others. They can nurture their inner child and begin healing these old wounds, laying the groundwork for healthier self-acceptance and empowerment.

Healthy self-acceptance requires authentic self-love. We learn to accept and appreciate ourselves unconditionally when we heal our inner child. For example, someone who experienced rejection in their formative years might have developed a harsh inner critic. This critical voice frequently undermines their self-esteem and prevents them from pursuing their dreams. But as you reparent yourself, you offer the support, encouragement, and validation that was lacking in your youth. It empowers you to silence your inner critic and embrace your authentic self with confidence and love.

Nourishing the inner child often reignites creativity and joy. Childlike wonder and creativity are buried under layers of adult responsibilities and societal expectations, but engaging in inner child work allows individuals to reconnect with their playful and imaginative side. It can lead to better mental health and fulfillment. Just like when kids lose themselves in play, adults who nurture their inner child often find a renewed sense of passion and excitement for life. Activities such as painting, dancing, or even playing games can help unlock this dormant creativity and provide immense joy and satisfaction.

Childhood traumas frequently result in maladaptive coping mechanisms that continue into adulthood. For instance, a person who experienced neglect may have developed a tendency to isolate themselves emotionally to avoid further pain. However, these coping strategies can be counterproductive in adult life, resulting in issues like anxiety or depression. Addressing and healing these childhood wounds helps us develop healthier ways to cope with stress and adversity, which increases resilience and adaptability, even when we face difficulties.

Say Hello to Your Inner Child

Have you started to see the child within you? It plays a vital role in understanding how childhood experiences shape your emotional health and behaviors as an adult. Our early experiences leave a lasting impact and influence everything from our self-esteem to our coping mechanisms. Patience, self-compassion, and frequent professional guidance are all necessary to heal the inner child. When you put in the work, you develop a deeper connection with yourself and increase your capacity to build fulfilling relationships and live a more balanced, joyful life. As you continue your exploration, remember that healing is a process, and each step you take brings you closer to emotional freedom and self-love.

2

Identifying Childhood Traumas

Childhood trauma isn't always loud and visible; sometimes, it appears quietly through emotional neglect or erupts violently through physical abuse. The aftermath of these experiences can linger for years and influence how we perceive ourselves and interact with the world around us. Recognizing these forms of trauma helps to map out the path they have carved into our sense of self and worth, often leading to behaviors and patterns that impede personal growth and healthy relationships.

Emotional Neglect vs. Physical Abuse

Childhood trauma can take many forms, each affecting a person's emotional and psychological well-being. Emotional neglect—when a child's emotional needs are consistently unmet by their caregivers—is a major concern. Emotional neglect can be subtle and challenging to identify, but it's characterized by the lack of attention, validation, and love that a child requires to develop a healthy sense of self-worth. Without the necessary emotional support, they may grow up feeling invisible, unworthy, and disconnected from their feelings. These invisible wounds can become part of a person's fiber and appear as chronic low self-esteem or an inability to recognize and express emotions.

Emotional Dysregulation

Another significant type of childhood trauma is physical abuse, which is the intentional infliction of harm on a child. For example, hitting, kicking, or other forms of violence. The visible scars from physical abuse are evident and unmistakable, but the deeper, less visible psychological scars left by physical abuse can have long-lasting implications. Children who endure physical abuse often struggle with immense feelings of fear, betrayal, and worthlessness. These emotions can heavily impact their self-esteem and determine how they interact with others throughout their lives.

Both emotional neglect and physical abuse can lead to emotional dysregulation. Children who experience these forms of trauma may find it challenging to deal with their emotions effectively, and this can continue into adulthood. Emotional dysregulation appears in various ways, such as intense mood swings, difficulty coping with stress, or a tendency to overreact to minor frustrations. Adults who were emotionally neglected or physically abused as children might struggle to maintain stable moods and may find it difficult to have healthy relationships. They might exhibit behavior patterns that come from their unresolved traumas, like avoiding intimacy, being overly dependent on others, or displaying aggression.

Childhood trauma shows up in adult behaviors in unique and diverse ways. For instance, adults who experienced emotional neglect might have trouble trusting others and could isolate themselves to avoid being hurt again. On the other hand, those who experienced physical abuse may develop a heightened sensitivity to perceived threats and react defensively in situations where they feel vulnerable. These defense mechanisms were developed during childhood as survival strategies, but they can prevent the formation of real connections and personal growth.

Reflect on Childhood Experiences

Take some time to reflect on your personal experiences of childhood trauma; it's a necessary step toward healing. By consciously acknowledging the specific forms of trauma you endured—whether emotional neglect or physical abuse—you can begin to understand the impact of these experiences on your life. The idea is not to blame yourself or others but to understand and validate your past to heal. Reflection can involve journaling, therapy, or participating in discussions within supportive communities. All of these options provide safe spaces for you to explore your past, express your emotions, and work through the pain associated with your childhood experiences.

Even though it's difficult, reflecting on emotional neglect helps you realize how a lack of emotional support shapes your self-perception and interactions. It allows you to acknowledge feelings of worthlessness that come from being emotionally ignored. This awareness can change everything because it empowers you to look for the emotional nurturing and validation you lacked in childhood from healthier sources in adulthood. Once you understand the insidious nature of emotional neglect, you start to equip yourself with the tools to break the cycle for future generations, ensuring that your own children receive the emotional support they need to thrive.

Reflecting on physical abuse enables you to confront the fear and powerlessness you felt as a child. Through this process, you can start to reclaim your sense of safety and autonomy, particularly because you are in control. It's essential to recognize that while physical abuse involves clear instances of harm, the psychological effects can be more complex and enduring. The invisible scars can last a lifetime, but working through these experiences in therapy or support groups can help you rebuild a sense of trust and security, which is crucial for forming healthy relationships.

Overlapping Child Traumas

You may have been exposed to one type of abuse or various kinds. The overlap between different forms of childhood trauma is important because all types of neglect and abuse disrupt the normal development of trust and attachment in children. Consequently, forming secure and healthy relationships becomes a challenge in adulthood. You might find yourself either excessively clinging to others for fear of abandonment or pushing people away for fear of getting hurt. It's important to recognize these patterns as consequences of past traumas so that you can address and modify these behaviors for healthier interpersonal connections.

Part of your healing journey should include developing strategies to manage emotional dysregulation. Techniques like mindfulness, cognitive behavioral therapy (CBT), and self-compassion exercises can be helpful. Mindfulness practices help you become aware of your emotions without judgment and allow you to respond thoughtfully rather than react impulsively. CBT helps to identify and challenge negative thought patterns related to self-worth and trauma. Meanwhile, self-compassion exercises help you to be kind toward yourself, creating a positive self-image and making you more emotionally resilient. We'll discuss all of these techniques in later chapters.

Adding these practices to your daily routines enables gradual healing and strengthens emotional regulation. It's also beneficial to educate yourself about the long-term impacts of childhood trauma on your mental health. Resources like books, articles, and support groups can give you valuable insights and validation. But remember, you are not alone: Others have successfully worked through similar experiences, and their stories offer hope and motivation.

Impact of Parental Relationships

Your relationship with your parents or guardians had an impact on shaping your emotional landscape as a child.

Different parenting styles have different effects on attachment patterns, which play a role in a child's ability to form healthy relationships later in life. Attachment theory shows that early interactions with caregivers shape how we view and engage in relationships later in life. Children with secure attachments tend to have better emotional stability and social skills, which is linked to better emotional regulation and good mental health. For example, secure attachment, characterized by consistent and responsive caregiving, develops resilience and equips children with the confidence to explore their environments and build positive relationships. In contrast, avoidant or anxious attachments result from inconsistent or unresponsive caregiving, which may lead to difficulties creating intimate connections in adulthood.

Role-Modeling Behavior

Parents are a child's primary role models, and their behaviors directly influence their children's actions and self-perceptions. Parents who display healthy coping mechanisms and conflict-resolution skills provide their children with a good example to emulate. Conversely, parental conflicts and negative behaviors can instill harmful beliefs about self-worth and love. For instance, parents who frequently argue or demonstrate hostile behavior may inadvertently teach their children that these interactions are normal. The children may then replicate this behavior in their future relationships.

Communication and Conflict Resolution

Healthy communication within the family is crucial for emotional well-being. Open, honest, and compassionate communication creates a sense of security and understanding among family members and allows children to express their needs and emotions without fear of judgment or retribution. On the other hand, poor communication can create misunderstandings and emotional estrangement. Children raised in environments where communication is lacking or dysfunctional may struggle to express their feelings and needs, which may lead to unresolved emotions and strained relationships in their adult lives.

For example, a child who grows up in a household where emotions are not openly discussed may internalize their feelings and bottle up unresolved emotions. As an adult, they may find it challenging to communicate effectively in their relationships and perpetuate a cycle of emotional disconnection and misunderstanding.

Unresolved conflicts with parents often manifest as relational patterns in adulthood. Children who frequently see their parents fight without resolving the issue may grow up believing that conflict is either unavoidable or unsolvable. This belief can hinder their ability to manage conflicts in their own relationships. However, addressing these unresolved conflicts can help a person to heal and break the cycle of dysfunctional relational patterns. Therapy, open conversations, and the implementation of healthy boundaries are all effective strategies to help address these conflicts.

Adverse Childhood Experiences (ACEs) Scale

An important tool to understand and heal from childhood trauma is the Adverse Childhood Experiences (ACEs) scale.

The ACEs framework categorizes various forms of childhood trauma and links them to chronic health issues and life patterns. This can help you better understand your past and its impact on your present.

The ACEs framework identifies 10 specific types of childhood trauma, including abuse, neglect, and household dysfunction. Examples include physical, emotional, and sexual abuse, as well as witnessing domestic violence or living with family members who have substance use disorders or mental illness. The structured approach emphasizes the varied nature of experiences that can impact long-term health. It makes it clear that trauma isn't limited to extreme cases but often includes more subtle yet equally damaging situations.

Through categorization, the ACEs framework allows you to see the connections between childhood adversity and adult health outcomes. Higher ACE scores are associated with an increased risk of chronic diseases such as heart disease, diabetes, and depression, which demonstrates why recognizing and addressing childhood trauma is necessary to prevent long-term health issues (Centers for Disease Control and Prevention, 2024).

The ACE Score

The ACE score is a tally of different types of adverse experiences endured before the age of 18. You can search for the ACE test online and complete the following steps to help you better understand your childhood and its impact on your life now.

1. Review each of the 10 questions related to abuse, neglect, and household dysfunction.

2. Answer each question honestly based on your experiences before turning 18.

3. For each "yes" answer, give yourself 1 point.

Research shows a dose-response relationship between the number of ACEs and adverse health outcomes. Individuals with an ACE score of 4 or more are at a much higher risk for issues such as depression, anxiety, substance abuse, and even suicide attempts (CDC, 2024). With this in mind, you can seek help and develop coping strategies to live a fulfilling life.

The ACE score does not measure your worth or future potential, but it can help you understand your personal history. Accepting these experiences is the first step toward healing since high ACE scores are connected to mental health challenges and strained relationships. Keep in mind that high scores do not doom you to a life of struggle; instead, resilience and support systems play a role in overcoming the impacts of ACEs.

Reflective Exercises

The ACEs scale forces you to reflect on personal experiences, but it's essential to do so non-judgmentally. You have to acknowledge what happened without assigning blame or shame and understand that the events were beyond your control. The focus should be on how your experiences have shaped current behaviors and feelings. Reflective exercises can be an invaluable part of this process. Simple journaling prompts like, "How do my childhood experiences affect my reactions today?" can uncover deep insights.

Reflective exercises make you accountable for progress during the healing process. Writing about specific memories and how they relate to current emotional responses takes time, but that can bring clarity and a sense of agency. For instance, if you realize your intense fear of abandonment stems from childhood neglect, you can work towards forming healthier attachments and communication patterns in your relationships. You may be able to recognize patterns that perpetuate pain and suffering and begin to break free from them. It creates self-compassion and empathy for yourself, which are critical parts of healing. It encourages you to take responsibility for your healing journey rather than remaining stuck in the victim mindset.

The connection between ACEs and adult behavior can also help you find more tailored and effective therapeutic approaches. Mental health practitioners can use the ACEs framework to better understand your history and to develop a treatment plan that suits your needs. This might include cognitive behavioral therapy, mindfulness practices, or other interventions to address the root cause of your trauma.

While high ACE scores indicate a greater risk for various problems, they also allude to the potential for resilience. Many people with high ACE scores go on to lead fulfilling, successful lives, especially once they better understand their inner child. Supportive relationships, positive self-perception, and opportunities for skill-building and education are some ways to build resilience. These techniques will be discussed in greater detail later on.

Long-Term Emotional Consequences

The emotional consequences of unhealed childhood trauma can endure long into adulthood. Many adults find themselves triggered by seemingly mundane events, unaware that these reactions are rooted in past traumatic experiences. It demonstrates the long-lasting impact of childhood trauma and why it needs to be addressed effectively.

Understanding Emotional Triggers

It helps to identify common triggers, such as specific sounds, scents, or situations, so you can better manage your emotional responses and begin disconnecting from those past traumas. Everyday triggers can range from a tone of voice reminding you of a critical parent to the smell of a particular food that brings up a distressing event. If you are aware of these triggers, you can start to anticipate and prepare for situations that might provoke intense emotional responses. This awareness allows you to consciously choose how to react rather than unconsciously falling into old patterns. For example, if you grew up with unpredictable caregivers, you may feel alarmed by sudden changes in plans. When you acknowledge this link, you can use coping strategies, like deep breathing or grounding exercises, to stay composed.

Cycles of Behavior

Unconscious habits may come from unresolved childhood trauma and be recreated in adult relationships. For example, you may consistently choose partners resembling emotionally unavailable caregivers or react to conflicts with undue intensity. Breaking these patterns requires better awareness of your unconscious choices and behaviors. For instance, a person who experienced abandonment as a child may unconsciously look for relationships where they can play out this dynamic, either by becoming overly dependent on their partner or pushing them away to avoid being abandoned. To disrupt this cycle, they have to cultivate self-awareness. Practices like reflective journaling, therapy, and mindfulness can help you recognize these repetitive patterns and make deliberate efforts to respond differently.

Emotional Dysregulation

Trauma survivors are often more sensitive to stress, resulting in extreme emotional responses. For instance, someone who witnessed frequent family arguments may react to disagreements with extreme anxiety or anger. They need to find strategies to manage emotions effectively to prevent these trauma responses from dominating their life. Skills such as emotional labeling, which involves identifying and naming your feelings, can diminish the power of these responses. Techniques like cognitive restructuring—where you challenge and change unhelpful thought patterns—also help in managing intense emotions. Relaxation methods such as yoga, meditation, or progressive muscle relaxation can help regulate your emotions and make it easier to deal with challenging situations without going back to trauma-induced reactions.

How It Affects Self-Identity

A common experience among trauma survivors is internalized negative self-talk. For example, a person who was frequently criticized as a child might grow up believing they are inherently inadequate. Unresolved trauma can skew your self-identity and worth. You may have limiting beliefs about yourself and feel unworthy, flawed, or incapable. Reflection exercises that challenge these beliefs can be helpful in creating positive self-reinforcement and a healthier self-image. You can list personal strengths or achievements to counteract these limiting beliefs. Cognitive-behavioral strategies, like replacing negative self-statements with positive affirmations, further reinforce a healthier self-concept. Approach the reflection process with kindness and patience.

Self-compassion is about treating yourself with the same kindness and care you would offer a friend. It means acknowledging your suffering without judgment and understanding that imperfections and mistakes are part of the human experience. Some ideas for practicing self-compassion are doing mindful self-care routines like taking time for enjoyable activities, taking a warm bath, or nature walks, which all help to nurture self-love and acceptance. Another option is to write letters to your younger self where you express understanding and empathy for past struggles. Similarly, you can have a conversation with your inner child, offering reassurance and validation, to help heal and rediscover your self-worth.

Common Triggers That Bring Back Past Trauma

We've already touched on triggers, but we need to take a closer look at them. An emotional trigger is something—like a word, memory, or situation—that evokes strong emotions like happiness, sadness, anger, or fear. These triggers usually remind you of past experiences and can affect how you act or feel in the moment.

Sensory Triggers

Many common triggers go back to unresolved childhood traumas from various sensory experiences. These sensory triggers may include sights, sounds, and smells that unexpectedly tap into stored memories. For instance, a specific type of music or song might take you back to a moment tied to intense emotions from your childhood. Familiar scents such as perfumes, foods, or even environmental odors like cut grass or rain-soaked earth can bring up strong emotional responses because they are linked to important events from your past. You need to be able to recognize these sensory triggers if you want to better manage the feelings they evoke.

Situational Triggers

Specific scenarios that remind you of conflicts or abandonment during childhood can trigger powerful emotional reactions. For example, being critiqued at work could mirror the scolding received from a parent and bring forth feelings of inadequacy and rejection. Additionally, being left alone or experiencing a breakup can amplify fears of abandonment rooted in childhood. A heightened awareness of situational triggers can help you prepare for and decrease emotional responses when you encounter similar situations in adulthood.

Interpersonal Triggers

Interpersonal triggers arise when you interact with people whose behaviors are similar to those of key figures from your past. For example, interactions with authority figures may rekindle feelings of helplessness experienced by a controlling parent. In another scenario, relationships with emotionally unavailable partners can re-open old wounds related to neglect. Establishing boundaries is indispensable when it comes to interpersonal triggers. Clear boundaries allow for safe and open expressions of needs and desires, which reduces the likelihood of reactivating past trauma-based patterns.

Emotional Triggers

Unresolved traumas can appear as emotional reactions to present-day experiences you perceive as threatening.

Identifying emotional triggers is a bit more challenging, but it is possible. Journaling is an effective tool as it is a structured way to explore and express your feelings. You can document your thoughts and emotions regularly to identify recurring patterns and connect present triggers with past traumas.

Self-compassion techniques are equally important to regulate emotional responses. When a traumatic memory resurfaces, it brings with it a flood of negative self-perceptions and emotions, but self-compassion, simple affirmations, and gentle self-talk can help soothe your inner critic and diminish the intensity of the emotional response.

Mindfulness practices further help with emotional regulation by grounding you in the present moment. Techniques like deep breathing, meditation, and body scans can help you observe and accept the sensations without judgment. Mindfulness allows you to pause and assess your response rather than reacting impulsively. Over time, this mindful approach increases your resilience, allowing for a more balanced and measured reaction to triggers.

It's also a good idea to get professional support to help you heal from childhood trauma. Working with a therapist or counselor trained in trauma-informed care offers a safe environment to unpack complex emotions and memories, even those you buried deep or don't want to share with other people. Therapists can suggest techniques like eye movement desensitization and reprocessing (EMDR) or cognitive behavioral approaches to process and reframe traumatic experiences. These therapeutic interventions assist in managing triggers and pave the way for long-term recovery.

Support groups are another option, and they provide a layer of healing through shared experiences and collective empathy. Being part of a community where others understand and relate to your struggles can be incredibly validating. Sharing stories and coping strategies within these groups builds a network of support that reinforces your positive changes and growth. The feeling of connection decreases the isolation you may feel from your trauma, which can give you a sense of belonging and acceptance.

Learning to identify and manage triggers requires patience and perseverance. You must incorporate this practice into daily life and develop a supportive framework to deal with challenges tied to your unresolved childhood trauma. Sensory, situational, and interpersonal triggers are inevitable parts of life, but you can reduce their impact with awareness and appropriate tools.

Reflect on Your Situation

Childhood trauma often leaves invisible wounds that leave you with feelings of unworthiness and disconnection from your emotions. These experiences have a long-lasting impact on your emotional and physical well-being. It shapes your interactions and self-esteem. Through reflection and by identifying these impacts, you can begin to see how your challenges with emotional regulation, relationship dynamics, and self-worth are rooted in these past experiences. Self-awareness and understanding can help you as you recover and enable you to break free from harmful patterns so that you can build healthier relationships in the present.

3

Assess Your Emotional Health

Your emotional health can tell you a lot about your inner child, especially the areas that need nurturing. It requires a process of self-discovery to understand your current emotional state better. You can use various self-assessment tools and techniques to get valuable insights into your emotional patterns, which helps you recognize triggers and recurring themes in your responses. Based on your observations, various tools and techniques are available to help you cope. But first, you have to get to grips with your emotions throughout your day so you can build a comprehensive picture of your emotional landscape. In turn, this will help you find your path toward healing from past traumas and better ongoing emotional health.

Self-Assessment Tools and Techniques

An important step in understanding yourself and identifying areas that may need healing is to assess your emotional health. Self-assessment methods offer valuable insights into your current emotional state and help track your progress over time.

Journaling Prompts

Journaling is a great way to gauge your emotional health as you answer thought-provoking questions that guide you to discover your feelings and triggers. Some potential prompts include:

- What emotions did I experience today?

- What events triggered these emotions?

- How did my body respond to these emotions?

- Are there any recurring themes in my emotional responses?

Regularly working through these prompts can give you a space for honest self-reflection so you have a greater awareness of your emotions. Try to go through them every few days but especially if you feel emotional. This practice helps you identify patterns and makes it easier to express feelings that might otherwise remain hidden.

Emotion Checklists

Emotion checklists are another valuable tool for self-assessment. Typically, these lists include a broad range of emotions, allowing you to pinpoint what you are currently feeling. To use an emotion checklist, you might start by marking all the emotions you've felt throughout the day and repeat this process for several days at a time. Over time, this exercise can reveal trends and fluctuations in your emotional state.

Emotion checklists can be beneficial when you struggle to express your feelings. Seeing a variety of emotions written down may make it easier to recognize and name what you're experiencing. Consistently using an emotion checklist can alert you to continuous negative emotions, which may indicate areas to explore further or even where you may need some kind of intervention.

Life Satisfaction Surveys

Life satisfaction surveys provide a comprehensive view of how different aspects of your life contribute to your overall emotional health. Usually, these surveys ask you to rate your satisfaction across various areas of your life, including relationships, work, leisure activities, and personal growth. The surveys use a numerical scale. For example, you might rate your satisfaction with your social connections or work satisfaction on a scale from 1 to 10.

Satisfaction surveys are a structured way to assess where you feel fulfilled and where you might feel lacking. They help you recognize the areas where you need to make targeted efforts to improve your quality of life. For instance, if you find low satisfaction in your career, you could explore opportunities for professional development or consider a career change to better align with your passions and skills. Similarly, you may find low scores in emotional areas or your relationships with family members, which could indicate a hurt inner child.

Mood Tracking Apps

Technology has made it much easier to keep track of various things, and that includes your mood. Mood-tracking apps are powerful tools to monitor daily emotional fluctuations and enable you to log your mood at different times of the day. It provides you with a visual representation of your emotional trends. Many of these apps also offer features like journaling spaces, reminders for regular check-ins, and even integration with other wellness tools such as meditation guides. Together, these different tools can give you a more holistic approach to healing your inner child and a more emotionally balanced life.

For example, the Mind Journal app is designed to help users understand their emotions through CBT techniques. It offers a mood tracker diary, guided reflection prompts, and mindfulness exercises to improve overall emotional health. Using an app like this can give you immediate insights into patterns and potential triggers for both positive and negative emotions. If you prefer a structured approach to self-assessment, these digital tools can be incredibly useful. They also become valuable records to share with a therapist or coach because they offer concrete data on your emotional journey.

Identifying Emotional Pain Points

Understanding and dealing with emotional wounds from childhood is an important part of healing and personal growth. These wounds can manifest as difficulty expressing emotions, low self-esteem, a harsh inner critic, or fear of abandonment and commitment issues. These patterns can shed light on the areas where your inner child needs nurturing and support.

Personal Reflection Exercises

An effective way to begin this process is through personal reflection exercises designed to help uncover deep-seated emotional pain. It prompts honest exploration of your emotions and experiences. For instance, you can dedicate time to writing about specific memories from your childhood to reveal recurring emotional themes. It's a great time to reflect on pivotal moments like family changes or significant losses and how they made you feel. As you examine these events, you can begin see how past experiences shape your current emotional state. Approach this process with compassion and understand that these reflections are not about placing blame but about gaining insight and awareness.

Trigger Analysis

A practical method to further understand your emotional wounds is through trigger analysis. Triggers are events, situations, or people that create strong emotional reactions. It can be challenging to identify your triggers, but it is an empowering step towards healing. Start by paying attention to moments when your emotional response seems disproportionately intense. Ask yourself why this is the case. Questions like the following can help: What exactly happened? Who was involved? Where were you, and what time was it? How did you feel immediately after? Does this situation remind you of any past events? This process helps to create connections between your present reactions and past experiences, specifically from childhood, which offers a clearer picture of unresolved emotional issues. It can be helpful to take note of these triggers and their emotional impact by writing them in your journal or a tracking app so that you can identify any recurring patterns.

Feedback From Others

Feedback from people you trust is another tool to help you recognize childhood emotional wounds. Close friends or family often observe aspects of your emotional behavior that you might overlook. Some of these people may have known you since childhood and seen events first-hand even though they couldn't intervene at that stage. Have open conversations with these trusted figures to get a different perspective, as they can highlight emotional patterns you may not have been aware of. It's important to choose supportive and non-judgmental people to ensure that their feedback is constructive. For example, ask them if they've noticed recurring themes in your reactions or if there are specific situations where you seem particularly emotionally charged. If they have specific examples, that can be useful to understand your behavior better. Other people's observations act as a mirror and reflect parts of your emotional world that need attention and nurturing.

Visualization

Visualizing emotional pain is a transformative technique that involves mapping out emotional pain points through art or diagrams to make abstract feelings more tangible. When you create visual representations of your emotions, it provides a new way of understanding and processing your experiences. For instance, draw a timeline of your life and mark significant emotional events to represent periods of turmoil and peace visually. Visualization can clarify how certain events influenced your emotional development. Visual aids like mind maps, flowcharts, or even expressive artwork can give you insights into how your past wounds affect your current state.

Role of Emotional Resilience

Emotional resilience is a huge part of your ability to heal from past trauma and effectively work through life's challenges. Emotional resilience is the capacity to adapt to stressful situations and bounce back from adversity. It does not mean avoiding stress or pain but focusing on how you can manage these experiences constructively. Being emotionally resilient allows you to face setbacks with strength and perseverance. It means you are able to maintain some level of functioning and emotional stability even in difficult times, which reduces the risk of developing mental health issues like depression and anxiety. The essence of emotional resilience lies in recognizing that life will have its ups and downs, and what's important is how you respond to these fluctuations.

It takes some time to develop emotional resilience, but it can make a significant difference as you heal and prioritize your emotional well-being. The importance of emotional resilience becomes apparent when you consider its impact on mental health. People with high levels of resilience are better equipped to handle both everyday stresses and major life crises. They can adapt more easily, use healthier coping mechanisms, and keep a positive outlook despite challenges (Sonu et al., 2024). This adaptability can be learned and strengthened over time because many people do not have it innately.

Resilience-Building Exercises

Think of building emotional resilience as if you were strengthening a muscle in your body; it requires consistent practice and effort. You can use several exercises and techniques to improve your emotional strength:

- **Mindfulness and Meditation**: Mindfulness helps you stay grounded in the present moment and reduces the tendency to ruminate on past traumas. Meditation, deep breathing exercises, and guided imagery can help you manage stress and bring about a sense of inner peace.

- **Journaling**: Write about your thoughts and feelings to process and release pent-up emotions effectively. Journaling allows you to reflect on your experiences, recognize patterns in your emotional responses, and develop healthier perspectives.

- **Positive Affirmations**: Repeat positive statements about yourself to counteract negative self-talk and build self-esteem. For example, you can include affirmations like "I am strong," "I can handle this," and "I am worthy of love."

- **Physical Activity**: Exercise is a great way to improve your mood and resilience. Activities like yoga, running, or even a gentle walk can help reduce stress and increase your overall well-being. Regular physical activity releases endorphins, which naturally improve your mood.

- **Social Support**: Build and maintain strong relationships with friends and loved ones for emotional support during tough times. Consider participating in community activities, joining support groups, or volunteering to help create a network of resilience-boosting connections.

- **Cognitive Reframing**: This technique is about changing how you think about challenges and setbacks. Instead of viewing them as overwhelming obstacles, learn to see them as opportunities for growth and learning. Cognitive reframing can significantly alter your emotional response to negative events and your inner child, empowering you to take proactive steps.

- **Resilience Training Programs**: Structured programs or workshops have been designed to help you build resilience, so attending one of them can be highly beneficial. These programs use evidence-based methods to teach skills like problem-solving, emotional regulation, and effective communication.

Stories of Resilience

Hearing about others' journeys through adversity and healing their inner child can be incredibly inspiring and reassuring. For example, Jane overcame severe childhood neglect by focusing on building her emotional resilience. She found solace in journaling and mindfulness practices, which helped her process her traumatic experiences. Jane also joined a local support group where she connected with others who had similar backgrounds and where they could share how they overcame their traumas. Over time, these practices increased her emotional strength and allowed her to lead a fulfilling and balanced life.

Another powerful story is that of Michael, who faced the scars of childhood trauma head-on. He knew he couldn't change his past, but he wanted to have a better future and help other people who might be experiencing similar struggles. Instead of allowing his past to dictate his future, Michael chose to use his inner strength for good. He began mentoring at a local youth center, which filled his time purposefully and helped him forge meaningful connections. Michael also turned to physical activity and therapy to nurture his mental well-being. Ultimately, he discovered a new life direction that brought him greater fulfillment than he had ever known before.

Stories like these demonstrate that while the path to resilience may be challenging, it is certainly attainable. Learning from real-life examples provides hope and practical insights that can help build your resilience. All you need to do is be open to different ideas and coping mechanisms, which you may be able to use in your own life, too.

Identify Your Strengths

A key component of building resilience is recognizing and using your personal strengths. First, you need to identify your strengths, and then you can use them in times of adversity, especially since you know that these are the good traits that make you feel better about yourself.

Here are some ways to find your strengths:

- **Strength Assessment Tools**: Various tools and questionnaires are available that can help pinpoint your inherent strengths. For example, the VIA Character Strengths survey categorizes strengths such as creativity, kindness, and perseverance. A quick online search should help you find some of these surveys.

- **Reflective Practices**: Spend time reflecting on past experiences where you successfully overcame challenges. What qualities did you exhibit? Were you particularly resourceful, patient, or assertive? By identifying these attributes, you can consciously rely on them in future stressful situations. It helps to write them down somewhere—like in a journal—so you can find them easily in difficult times.

- **Feedback from Others**: Sometimes, other people see strengths in us that we might overlook. Ask your trusted friends, family members, or colleagues for their observations, as they can provide valuable insights into your strengths.

- **Strength Journaling**: Create a journal dedicated to capturing moments when you used your strengths. Reflect on how these strengths helped you deal with specific situations and how they can be applied to ongoing and future challenges.

- **Goal Setting**: Set goals that align with your strengths. For instance, if creativity is one of your strengths, find ways to incorporate creative tasks into your daily routine. This alignment can increase your resilience and positively impact your overall life satisfaction.

- **Visualization Techniques**: Visualization can be a potent tool for resilience. Imagine scenarios where you effectively use your strengths to overcome obstacles, especially as you work through childhood trauma. This mental rehearsal prepares you for real-life scenarios and strengthens your confidence.

Understand Your Emotional Patterns

As part of assessing your emotional health, you need to recognize recurring emotional behaviors and patterns that developed in response to your childhood experiences. These patterns often emerge as a way of coping with adverse events and can continue into adulthood, shaping your responses in various situations. Past behaviors can give you valuable insight into the lasting impact of your early experiences and help you identify areas where you can improve.

Pattern Recognition Techniques

Observing and recording your emotional responses over time is a great way to recognize recurring emotional patterns. For example, you can keep an emotion journal. Each day, take a few minutes to jot down your feelings, the situations that triggered them, and any subsequent reactions. Over time, you should be able to spot trends and identify consistent emotional triggers.

Once again, mood-tracking apps can help, as these digital tools allow you to log your emotions at different points throughout the day. Many of these apps provide visual representations of your data, which makes it easier to spot patterns in your emotional responses. Reflective writing exercises can also help you uncover underlying themes in your emotions. Write about significant experiences and how they made you feel, but as you do, pay close attention to any recurring emotions or reactions that come up.

Linking Past to Present

Connecting your childhood experiences to your current emotional patterns requires introspection and guided activities. One option is to create a timeline of significant life events. List key moments from your childhood and reflect on the emotions associated with each event. Then, consider how these emotions appear in your present life. For instance, if you experienced abandonment as a child, examine whether you have a heightened sensitivity to rejection in adult relationships. This process can take time, so be patient and gentle with yourself.

Therapeutic techniques like inner child work can also be beneficial. For this exercise, visualize yourself as a child and address unresolved emotions or unmet needs from that time. Through compassionate dialogue with your younger self, you can begin to heal old wounds and change negative emotional patterns.

Guided imagery exercises are another method to explore connections between your past and present. Close your eyes and envision a specific childhood memory; allow yourself to experience all the emotions tied to that memory. Next, bring those feelings into your current situation and observe how they influence your reactions and behaviors today. This process should give you a deeper understanding of how your early experiences continue to shape your emotional reality.

Cognitive Distortions

Cognitive distortions are thinking mistakes that distort your perception of reality, often worsening your emotional distress (Garey, 2023). Common cognitive distortions include all-or-nothing thinking, overgeneralization, and emotional reasoning. All-or-nothing thinking involves viewing situations in black-and-white terms without recognizing the nuances. For example, believing that failing once as a child makes you a total failure exemplifies this distortion.

Overgeneralization occurs when you draw broad conclusions based on limited evidence. A single negative event leads to the belief that similar outcomes will always follow. For instance, being abandoned as a child can make you believe that people will always abandon you. Emotional reasoning is about accepting your emotions as facts without questioning their validity. Feeling inadequate, for instance, might lead to the incorrect assumption that you are inherently flawed.

You need to learn to identify and challenge these cognitive distortions so you can improve your emotional health. Start by noticing when you engage in distorted thinking. Ask yourself whether your thoughts are based on facts or emotions. Reframe your negative thoughts by looking for evidence that contradicts your initial ideas. For example, if you think you're a failure because of one mistake, reflect on past successes to balance your perspective.

Behavioral Patterns

Your coping strategies, developed in response to emotional distress, can greatly influence your behavior. It's crucial to analyze these strategies to determine whether they are adaptive or maladaptive. Adaptive strategies, like seeking social support or doing physical activities, improve your emotional well-being. In contrast, maladaptive strategies, like substance abuse or avoidance, can hinder your emotional growth. Begin by listing your common coping mechanisms and think about whether they are effective. Consider how each strategy impacts your emotional health in the long term. For example, while drinking alcohol may provide temporary relief from anxiety, it can lead to greater distress over time.

Mindfulness meditation is an excellent practice for becoming more aware of your coping behaviors. Focusing on the present moment and observing your thoughts and feelings without judgment can help you gain clarity on why you behave the way you do. This awareness creates space for you to choose healthier responses to emotional challenges. Similarly, CBT can also be highly beneficial because it focuses on identifying and modifying unhelpful thought patterns and behaviors. Through therapy, you can develop more constructive ways to deal with emotional distress. As you work through your coping strategies, determine which ones are serving you well (adaptive) and which ones you need to change (maladaptive) so you can build your strengths.

Healthy vs. Unhealthy Coping Mechanisms

Let's talk a bit more about adaptive and maladaptive coping strategies and how they impact your emotional health. Your coping strategies affect how you heal from childhood traumas and can empower you to make healthier choices in your daily life.

Characteristics of Healthy Coping

Healthy coping mechanisms are essential tools to manage stress and emotional turmoil. These strategies can help you address the root causes of your problems rather than merely masking symptoms. Adaptability is a key characteristic of healthy coping, as you need to evolve with changing circumstances so you can experience personal growth. For instance, mindfulness practices like meditation or deep-breathing exercises can help you stay grounded in the present moment, which may reduce anxiety and improve your mental clarity. Another hallmark of healthy coping is proactive problem-solving. You should be able to approach challenges with a clear plan and the determination to find solutions, reducing feelings of helplessness and giving you a sense of control over your life.

Healthy coping also requires a balanced lifestyle that includes regular physical activity, sufficient sleep, and a nutritious diet. Exercise, for example, is known to release endorphins, which are natural mood lifters. Hobbies and activities that bring joy and satisfaction can become healthy distractions and give your mind a break from stressors. Social support is another important aspect of healthy coping since good relationships offer emotional nourishment and practical assistance during difficult times. Reaching out to friends, family, or support groups can give you different perspectives and increase your resilience.

Identifying Unhealthy Coping Mechanisms

Maladaptive coping mechanisms often provide temporary relief, but they will exacerbate problems in the long run. The first step toward change is to recognize these behaviors. Substance abuse, for instance, is a common maladaptive strategy. Whether it's alcohol, drugs, or even excessive caffeine, relying on substances to numb pain can lead to addiction and additional health issues (Cortez et al., 2023). Avoidance is another maladaptive behavior. When faced with stress, some people choose to withdraw from social interactions or responsibilities, hoping the problem will resolve itself, but this approach usually results in unresolved issues piling up and creating even more stress.

Maladaptive coping can also appear in forms like excessive rumination or dwelling on negative thoughts. The constant replaying of stressful events keeps a person stuck in a cycle of negativity, which increases feelings of depression and anxiety (Thompson et al., 2010). Self-harm or reckless behaviors are more extreme forms of unhealthy coping. These actions can temporarily distract or relieve emotional pain but also cause serious physical harm and perpetuate a cycle of self-destructive behavior. Emotional eating, where individuals consume large quantities of food to cope with stress, often leads to weight gain and associated health problems, further complicating emotional well-being. These are just some examples of maladaptive coping mechanisms, but there are many others; that's why it's so important to log your coping strategies and assess their impact on your life.

Create a Coping Toolkit

A personalized coping toolkit can be an excellent step to improve your emotional health. The first guideline for building this toolkit is self-awareness. Identify what triggers your stress responses so that you can select appropriate coping strategies ahead of time. Journaling can help you identify your triggers. By writing down your thoughts and emotions, you can identify patterns and triggers, which make it easier to choose effective coping methods.

Next, brainstorm relaxation techniques you can use during stressful moments. Methods like progressive muscle relaxation or guided imagery can quickly reduce your stress levels. Including a variety of these techniques ensures that you have options when different situations arise. You can also make a list of physical activities that you enjoy, such as yoga, hiking, or dancing.

Social support networks are indispensable, so make a list of trustworthy contacts who can provide emotional or practical support during challenging times. Getting hold of them through text, a call, or in-person visits should be easy. Another part of your coping toolkit should be self-care. Activities like taking a warm bath, reading your favorite book, or spending time in nature can improve your emotional well-being. The practice of gratitude journaling—writing down things you are grateful for each day—can also enhance your outlook and increase resilience. Lastly, learn new skills or hobbies that can distract you from stressors while giving you an opportunity for personal growth.

The Role of Professional Support

Professional support can make a massive difference in adopting healthier coping strategies. Therapists and counselors are trained to help you explore your emotions, understand your coping mechanisms, and develop better approaches. Professional therapists and counselors have an objective perspective, so they can help you identify unhealthy patterns that might be invisible to you. CBT, for example, is highly effective in treating various forms of maladaptive coping by helping you reframe negative thinking patterns and develop constructive behaviors.

Coaches and therapists also provide structured environments where you can safely express your feelings without judgment. This safe space is critical for dealing with deeply rooted issues that may have been buried for years, even from childhood. Professional support often involves accountability. Regular sessions ensure that you continuously work toward your goals and refine your coping strategies. Techniques like role-playing and exposure therapy can help you confront your fears and build new, positive experiences that replace negative associations from past traumas. Mental health professionals can also help you develop a coping toolkit tailored to your needs by offering expert advice on specific strategies that align with your unique challenges and strengths.

Get to Know Your Emotional Health

Throughout this chapter, we have looked at various self-assessment tools and techniques to evaluate your emotional health. These tools can give you a better understanding of your emotional state and offer structured ways to reflect on your feelings, identify patterns, and recognize areas that need attention. With these insights, you can create a plan for targeted efforts and improvements in your well-being. As you move forward, remember that assessing your emotional health is an ongoing process. Emotions can fluctuate as they are influenced by many internal and external factors. Stay connected to your emotional state by using self-reflection tools regularly so you can make informed choices for your well-being. The path to healing and growth requires patience, self-compassion, and a commitment to continuous self-reflection, but it will make you a more resilient and emotionally balanced person.

BUILDING SELF-AWARENESS

Self-awareness, and building it, is an important part of your journey toward healing your inner child. Self-awareness gently invites you to observe the complexities of your inner world, shedding light on patterns that have quietly governed your life. When you connect with this deeper understanding of yourself, you tap into a source of insight that can guide you through emotional challenges. If you feel lost in your own thoughts and reactions, then this chapter is a map that can help you break free from the cycles you are stuck in. It's about finding those moments of clarity where everything seems to come into focus, even if just for a moment, and seizing them as opportunities for change and growth.

Mindfulness Practices and Their Benefits

We've already touched on mindfulness a few times, and it comes up once again as a tool to improve self-awareness. At its core, mindfulness is about staying present and fully engaged in the moment. It's about moving away from your mind and spiraling thoughts by focusing on what is happening around you. This practice can disrupt the cycles of negative thought patterns that often ensnare us and emphasizes observation without judgment. Think about mindfulness this way: You're at a riverbank, watching leaves drift by. Your thoughts are like these leaves—passing without needing to be plucked or held onto. This imagery shows how mindfulness allows us to observe our mental processes from a distance, which reduces their control over us.

Mindful Breathing Techniques

When dealing with trauma or challenging emotions, the simple act of mindful breathing helps to ground you. If you feel like you are caught in a storm of emotions, where everything feels overwhelming, mindful breathing becomes a refuge of calm amid this chaos. At a minimum, focus on your breath, slowly inhaling through the nose, and gently exhaling. While you do this, shift your attention from swirling ideas to the present moment. This intentional focus creates space between something that triggers you and your response, which allows for thoughtful rather than impulsive reactions. There are many other mindful breathing techniques you can look into. For now, set aside a few minutes each day to concentrate solely on breathing to cultivate patience and resilience over time.

Mindful Movement

Mindful movement is another way to nurture self-awareness. Activities like yoga or walking meditation combine physical and emotional experiences, so they become a method to release pent-up emotions. Yoga, for example, is an invitation to explore your bodily sensations and connect them to internal emotional states as you complete each pose. This combination creates an awareness of how stress or tension appears physically and gives you an opportunity to release that tension. On the other hand, walking meditation encourages attentiveness to each step and breath, reinforcing the harmony between your body and mind. These activities present a meditative rhythm that provides an emotional release and a chance for introspection. As you tune into your body's cues and movements, you may find clarity and insight into emotions previously buried beneath layers of trauma and day-to-day life.

Observation

Often, we might feel trapped by strong emotions or try to ignore them completely, even though we know they are lingering in the background. Mindfulness is about finding a balance where you acknowledge these feelings without getting stuck in them. Think of mindful observation as sitting quietly in a room full of mirrors, where each mirror shows different sides of your thoughts and feelings. They are just reflections, not who you truly are. This way of thinking decreases the hold these thoughts have on your actions and leads to kinder self-reflection. Instead of being hard on yourself, mindfulness focuses on a gentle approach that increases your understanding and acceptance of your emotions and situation.

Mindfulness can improve mental health and assist with recovery from issues like anxiety or depression. Regular mindfulness practice helps prevent relapses by keeping you focused on the present and reducing your worries about the past or future (National Institutes of Health, 2021). When you are mindful, instead of getting overwhelmed by thoughts like "Nothing ever works out for me," you learn to notice them without judgment. You observe them, and with time, this separation helps you choose better ways to respond.

Tips for Mindfulness

Starting mindfulness is simple. It begins with small steps, like taking a few moments to sit quietly each day or focusing on your breathing. A few minutes already makes a difference. As you become more comfortable, you can increase the time you spend doing mindful activities. The important part is to be consistent and patient. Like learning any new skill, mindfulness improves with regular practice.

Mindfulness doesn't require big changes or dramatic actions. It's about paying more attention to everyday moments instead of overlooking them. For example, you can enjoy your morning coffee more by really tasting it, listening closely when people talk, or noticing how the water feels during a shower. Mindfulness can turn ordinary activities into chances to connect with your feelings, mind, and body.

Reflective Journaling Exercises

Reflective journaling is a powerful tool if you want to increase your self-awareness and gain emotional insight, especially if you need to uncover emotions surrounding your experienced trauma or emotional neglect in childhood. Journaling provides a personal sanctuary where you can openly express and process challenging emotions.

It is a safe, judgment-free space where you can express feelings that may be difficult to articulate aloud. This process helps clarify your thoughts and emotions so that you can understand them better. For instance, by regularly jotting down emotions that arise during the day, you may spot a pattern that gives insights into your recurring feelings and reactions. Consistent reflection can help you demystify your emotions and allow you to deal with them more effectively.

Reflective Writing Prompts

Writing prompts can deepen this self-exploration. Prompts about specific questions or themes can help you uncover hidden layers of your psyche. Prompting questions might include reflections about childhood memories and how they influence your current behaviors. Exploring these memories through journaling can emphasize longstanding emotional responses and patterns, which deepens your self-awareness.

Here are some reflective questions and prompts to give you a starting point:

- Describe a specific memory from your childhood that still affects you today. How does it shape your feelings and behaviors now?

- What were your biggest fears as a child? Do you still carry any of those fears into your adult life?

- What activities or experiences brought you joy as a child? How can you reconnect with those moments today?

Review and Reflect

Look back at your past journal entries to see how your feelings have changed over time. This review helps you spot patterns, like ongoing doubts or fears, that come up in similar situations. Knowing about these patterns can help you find ways to deal with challenges and turn recurring problems into chances to grow. You can look back on how you dealt with certain feelings before so that you can be better prepared for similar situations in the future.

Develop a Journaling Routine

By now, you know that regular journaling is essential for self-discovery. Writing consistently helps with reflection and holding yourself accountable. Set aside time each day or week to make self-reflection a regular part of your routine instead of something you do occasionally. It will help you connect better with your thoughts and feelings, build self-discipline, and push you to face your emotions instead of hiding from them.

Pick a time when you feel relaxed, like in the morning or before bed, when you have a few minutes to reflect. Some people like to write down their thoughts after a long day to help them relax and think about what happened. The goal is to create a comfortable space where journaling feels like a natural part of your day.

If you're new to journaling, it's important to be aware of your expectations. You don't need to write beautifully or create long entries. Simply let your thoughts flow freely without worrying about how they sound. It's okay if you only write down a few words, and it's also okay if you seem to be writing pages at a time. Over time, this freedom can lead to deeper insights and realizations, and looking back at your entries can help you see how you've grown and changed.

Tracking Emotional Responses in Daily Life

Monitoring your daily emotions enables you to identify personal triggers that might otherwise remain hidden. When you consistently track your feelings, noticing subtle changes and patterns becomes easier. Your self-inquiry deepens as you question why certain emotions arise under particular circumstances. You'll be better prepared to manage your emotional responses as you gather more information about yourself.

Create an Emotional Log

An emotional log is a bridge between fleeting feelings and concrete awareness. It includes event details, emotions experienced, bodily sensations, and subsequent reactions. For instance, after a challenging meeting at work, you might record feeling anxious, with tightness in your chest, followed by a reaction of withdrawal or irritability. Later on, you might realize that this response is tied to academic pressure from your childhood. The process of logging changes abstract emotional experiences into something tangible that you can reflect on.

To ensure that tracking is effective, create a system that works for you. Consistency is key, whether you use a notebook, a mood-tracking app, or voice memos. Don't shy away from experimenting with different methods until you find the one that works best. Be candid and authentic in your entries; remember, this log is for you alone. Honesty will help you recognize patterns without the bias of judgment or shame.

Analyze Patterns

Review your logs every now and then to identify repetitive patterns or cycles of emotions linked to your past traumas or significant life events. You might notice how specific interactions trigger similar emotional responses, which brings awareness to unhealthy patterns you may want to change. Recognizing these cycles can help you pinpoint areas where you need healing or change.

Shift Your Responses

As you get to grips with your emotional triggers, you're empowering yourself to respond differently. Once you pinpoint what causes certain feelings, you can develop ways to handle them better. One important strategy is reframing thoughts. For example, instead of assuming you failed when you are criticized, see it as an opportunity for growth. A change in perspective can change your emotional outcomes and transform negativity into learning moments.

Another tactic is to pause before reacting. A brief break gives you time to process emotions and consider possible outcomes instead of responding impulsively. During this pause, do a calming activity like deep breathing or mindful observation to tone down intense emotions. Intentional actions improve your resilience and make it easier to choose healthier emotional responses over ingrained reactions.

It's a good idea to think about what specific emotions you are trying to communicate. Each emotion carries a message about your needs or values. Anxiety might signal the need for preparation, while anger could indicate a boundary being crossed. By tuning into these messages, you can become better at understanding yourself and your underlying needs, leading to better decision-making that aligns with your values and well-being.

Do not suppress or avoid your emotional responses, but focus on acknowledging and interpreting them constructively. The idea is to take control of your emotional state rather than being controlled by it. Engage with your emotions—both comfortable and uncomfortable—to better understand yourself. You can support yourself during emotionally charged times by offering empathy and compassion. Be gentle with yourself during difficult emotional periods and acknowledge your humanity and vulnerability. Everyone has complex feelings that aren't always easy to deal with, and that reminder can help you be kinder to yourself.

The Importance of Self-Reflection

Self-reflection is an integral part of personal growth and emotional healing, serving as an anchor toward self-awareness. When you evaluate your feelings, thoughts, and behaviors, self-reflection helps you understand their origins. It's a process that develops personal accountability and unlocks paths to growth by encouraging you to explore what's happening inside you.

It can be enlightening to reflect on certain emotions and why you react in specific ways. For example, if you have recurrent anger toward a family member, reflection may help you uncover past experiences or unresolved emotions influencing this pattern. Acknowledging these triggers allows you to change and offers insights into avoiding repetitive, harmful cycles. As your understanding evolves, so does your capacity for compassion toward yourself and others, which creates healthier relationships and emotional resilience.

Reflective Questions

Reflection questions are great tools for introspection as they connect important moments from the past with present realities. Reflective questions prompt you to consider what shaped your current beliefs and behaviors. Questions like "What do I want to change about my behavior?" or "What fears are holding me back?" encourage a deeper sense of self-exploration. These questions open a conversation with your past and shed light on choices influenced by old wounds. The hope is that self-reflection can help you break free from your past and lead to better decisions in the future.

Feedback Loops

A feedback loop is like a circle of information. When you do something and see the results, that feedback helps you decide what to do next. Feedback helps you evaluate your actions based on your experiences. For example, when you experience an emotion, such as sadness from a childhood memory, that feeling can lead to self-reflection. You might think about why that memory makes you sad, and this reflection can help you understand that the sadness comes from a feeling of loss or unmet needs from your childhood. With this understanding, you might choose to address these feelings by practicing self-compassion or doing activities that nurture your inner child. This positive change in how you respond can reduce the sadness and lead to feelings of healing and empowerment. This step-by-step process encourages good behavior changes and builds emotional strength to deal with future challenges. It's about learning from each experience to grow stronger and more adaptable.

Setting Intentions for Reflection

Clear goals for reflection help you focus your thoughts and turn insights into steps for personal growth. Reflection becomes something you do on purpose when you have a specific goal. Goals steer your reflections toward areas you need to work on and make them meaningful. For example, if you want to get better at communication, set a goal to think about your conversations to help you find areas where you struggle, like being more assertive. Over time, these reflections can create a habit that helps you grow every day.

To make your reflection deeper, come up with exploratory questions. Start by listing areas of your life you want to consider, like your relationships or healing your inner child. Come up with open-ended questions that push you to think differently and honestly. Questions like "What achievements am I most proud of?" or "How do my insecurities show up in my interactions?" help you to look beyond the surface. Regularly answering these questions can give you new insights and keep your growth on track. But be patient and kind to yourself because it can take time to find meaningful answers.

Create a Safe Space for Self-Exploration

A nurturing environment is crucial for self-discovery and healing, especially since you have experienced childhood trauma.

Establish a Safe Environment

The first step in creating a nurturing environment is to establish a safe space that allows you to express your emotions openly without fear of judgment or retribution. It should be a comforting and secure physical space that acts as a sanctuary for emotional honesty. When you have a safe space to remove the fears associated with vulnerability, you create an opportunity for deeply rooted issues to surface.

Physical spaces can greatly influence our mental state. A home or room designed with calming colors, comfortable furniture, and personal mementos supports emotional safety and helps ground you in the present moment. It becomes a retreat from the chaos of daily life where you can immerse yourself in introspection without distractions. In these spaces, your emotional barriers start to dissolve, making way for genuine self-reflection and growth. Take some time today to look at your surroundings and transform your living space into a haven of peace and security. Find some items that help you feel safe and keep those close in times of difficulty.

Practices to Nurture Safety

In addition to creating a physically secure environment, regular calming practices can improve your psychological safety. Practices like meditation, deep breathing exercises, or repeating affirmations bring a sense of peace and stability. They are gentle reminders of your right to feel and express emotions authentically. For instance, starting the day with positive affirmations like "I am worthy" or "I embrace my feelings" can set a compassionate tone for all your interactions and thoughts throughout the day. Spend a few minutes being mindful each day, or keep a journal where you freely express thoughts and feelings. Surround yourself with people who understand your journey, advocate for your growth, and are there to support you when needed.

Supportive Relationships

A supportive network is invaluable during this journey, especially since some people can become a safe space for you. Friends, family, or therapists who understand you and show empathy create external security. These relationships are built on trust and allow you to get to know yourself better because you know you have allies who will support you through your discoveries. Therapists, in particular, offer professional guidance, helping unravel complex emotions and providing insights that might be difficult to achieve alone. Friends and loved ones, meanwhile, offer solace and reassurance, validating experiences and emotions, which fosters openness.

Embody Self-Kindness

Being kind to yourself is part of creating a supportive environment to help fight off self-criticism. It's important to remember that everyone makes mistakes and faces difficulties, but instead of judging yourself harshly for what you've done wrong, you should treat those moments with understanding and care. Self-kindness means recognizing your struggles while keeping a positive inner dialogue. When negative thoughts pop up, saying things like "It's okay, I'm doing my best" can change how you feel inside.

Building a supportive environment takes time; it doesn't happen all at once. You want to surround yourself with positivity and compassion to better understand your emotions. Becoming more self-aware and healing requires patience, but every step forward is important, no matter how small it seems. As you learn to trust your surroundings and the people in your life, you open up to more profound self-discovery and healing. Be kind to yourself and spend time with supportive people to create a solid base for long-term emotional health. Each moment you spend taking care of yourself adds to your strength and ability to bounce back from difficulties.

Know Yourself

Self-awareness is part of the healing process and can become a huge part of your emotional recovery. Self-awareness can ground you during life's storms and help you learn to respond thoughtfully rather than impulsively.

By regularly recording your thoughts and feelings, patterns emerge that help you understand recurring behaviors and emotions, enabling you to identify triggers and develop strategies for healthier reactions. Self-awareness can make it easier to break free from limiting cycles. But you also want to establish an environment that is safe and conducive to self-discovery, including surrounding yourself with supportive individuals.

5

EMBRACE SELF-LOVE

Self-love is the practice of caring for and loving yourself. It requires you to develop habits and practices that nurture your well-being and heal your inner child. There are many ways to love yourself more, including positive affirmations, self-compassion, self-care, and spending time doing things that make you feel good. By regularly reinforcing empowering messages, you begin to counteract harmful narratives and create a supportive inner dialogue.

Positive Affirmations and Their Impact

Affirmations can help you reshape negative self-beliefs and encourage a loving relationship with yourself. Rooted in the power of positive thinking, affirmations are statements that reinforce your self-worth and help you create a positive self-image. These simple yet powerful tools can assist you in healing from trauma and emotional neglect.

Positive affirmations work by counteracting negative thoughts and beliefs about yourself. Phrases like "I am deserving of love," "I am capable," or "I am enough" can replace harmful narratives with empowering messages, especially if you repeat them frequently. These affirmations help shift your mindset from focusing on your perceived flaws and failures to recognizing your strengths and potential. Over time, you will develop a more supportive and compassionate inner dialogue to help heal emotional wounds and increase self-love.

Create Effective Affirmations

Crafting effective affirmations requires some thought and personalization. The affirmations should reflect your core values and aspirations. Personalized messages resonate more deeply because they speak directly to your unique experiences and desires. For instance, if one of your core values is resilience, you might craft an affirmation such as "I face challenges with courage and strength." This personalized statement reinforces your value of resilience and empowers you to see yourself as someone who confronts difficulties with confidence.

Another important aspect of crafting affirmations is using the present tense. Affirmations should be stated as if they are already true to help train your mind to accept them as reality. Instead of saying, "I will be confident," say, "I am confident." This subtle difference creates a sense of immediacy and certainty, which makes it easier for your mind to accept and internalize the positive message.

Add Affirmations to Your Day

Make time to use affirmations throughout your day to increase your chances of using them successfully. There are several ways to add affirmations seamlessly into your life. For example, visual reminders, such as sticky notes on your mirror or desk, can be constant prompts to recite your affirmations throughout the day. You can also set aside specific times, such as during your morning routine or before bed, to repeat affirmations. Using affirmations during challenging moments can be quite helpful because they give you a mental boost when you need it most.

Measure the Impact

Consider keeping a journal to track changes in your mindset and overall well-being to evaluate the effectiveness of affirmations. Write down your daily affirmations and reflect on any shifts in your thoughts and feelings to determine how this practice is impacting your life. You can also ask for feedback from trusted individuals, such as friends or a therapist, for external validation and encouragement. They may notice positive changes in your behavior and attitude that you might overlook, but their words also act as affirmations.

Self-affirmations can broaden a person's perspective and reduce the impact of negative emotions (Cascio et al., 2015). By focusing on core values and rewarding experiences, affirmations activate neural mechanisms (parts of the brain) associated with positive valuation and reward. It strengthens the reward system so that your brain craves the affirmations. This process improves your overall psychological well-being, makes you more resilient to stress, and better equips you to handle life's challenges.

Using affirmations frequently can lead to a healthier relationship with yourself. Regularly affirming your worth and capabilities can decrease the pervasive influence of negative self-talk and nurture a more loving and supportive inner conversation. As you deal with childhood trauma or emotional neglect, this shift in self-perception is important to break free from unhealthy patterns so that you can achieve emotional freedom.

The transformative power of affirmations has been proven before. Many people say they experienced a significant improvement in their self-esteem and outlook on life after adding affirmations into their daily routines (Cascio et al., 2015). For example, someone struggling with self-doubt might find that regularly telling themselves, "I am worthy of success," gradually builds their confidence and motivates them to pursue their goals with greater determination.

But it's also important to acknowledge that the impact of affirmations may vary from person to person. You may feel they work for you, while someone else believes they don't get much from affirmations. Similarly, how well they work can vary at different times in your life. Factors like the severity of your past trauma, current emotional state, and level of commitment to the practice can influence the outcomes. That's why it's crucial to approach affirmations with patience and an open mind, understanding that positive change may take time.

Self-Compassion vs. Self-Criticism

Self-compassion is about treating yourself with kindness and understanding during difficult times. This means viewing your flaws and mistakes as part of the human experience rather than beating yourself up over them. When you approach yourself with a gentle, supportive attitude, you create an environment for emotional healing and personal growth.

On the other hand, harsh self-critique often leads to feelings of shame and inadequacy. Berating yourself for not meeting certain expectations or making mistakes only deepens your emotional wounds from past traumas. This relentless internal criticism can be paralyzing and block any attempts at self-improvement because you become too afraid of failure or further criticism. It is essential to recognize that self-criticism increases negativity and reduces your ability to heal and grow.

Benefits of Self-Compassion

Self-compassion has benefits that go beyond just feeling good about ourselves. People who practice self-compassion are more resilient and build better relationships. Self-compassion also provides a sense of safety to admit our mistakes, accept responsibility, and learn from them without harsh self-judgment. In contrast to being self-critical, self-compassionate individuals are more likely to act in helpful ways and stay motivated, even after facing challenges. People who are kind to themselves tend to take more initiative and responsibility for their personal growth.

Instead of being motivated by fear or the approval of others, they follow their goals because they want to. They are less likely to procrastinate. Some people hurt their chances of success because they fear failure or worry that they won't meet the high standards set by themselves, but self-compassion counteracts this so that people are more gentle with themselves. It's also been proven that people who learned to be kinder to themselves felt less anger and anxiety when thinking about their mistakes. They also took more responsibility for their actions than those who were hard on themselves (Salzgeber, 2017).

How to Nurture Self-Compassion

There are several techniques to improve your self-compassion. One effective method is self-soothing practices, which include physical activities like taking a warm bath, going for a walk in nature, or practicing yoga, as well as mental and emotional exercises such as mindfulness meditation or writing a compassionate letter to yourself. It's important to create moments that calm and reassure you as it gives you a break from the cycle of self-judgment, offering space for recovery and reflection.

Reframing negative thoughts is another excellent technique. When you find yourself engaging in negative self-talk, acknowledge these thoughts without judgment and then gently challenge and replace them with more compassionate ideas. For example, if you find yourself thinking, "I'm such a failure for not completing that project on time," try reframing it to something kinder like, "I faced some challenges and did my best under the circumstances. I can learn from this experience and do better next time."

Comparing Self-Compassion and Self-Criticism

The difference between self-compassion and self-criticism becomes clear when we look at their long-term effects. Self-compassion helps people recover from tough times more easily. This ability to heal comes from feeling safe and supported, which makes it easier to deal with life's problems. On the other hand, self-criticism weakens this ability and leaves people open to feelings of shame and discouragement.

People who practice self-compassion often have better relationships. They are used to being kind to themselves, which sets an example of good behavior to others. They are more likely to be empathetic and understanding, resulting in stronger connections and a supportive community where emotional growth can happen. In contrast, self-criticism can cause relationship problems and lead to defensiveness, blame, and mistrust.

Start with small steps if you want to develop a more self-compassionate mindset. Identify times when you are hard on yourself and try to think of yourself in a kinder way. It takes some time to get used to this, but try your best to catch yourself when you have a negative or harsh thought. Be kind to yourself, do things that help you relax and care for yourself, and build the habit of seeing your worth, no matter your successes or failures. Remember, self-compassion doesn't mean ignoring your mistakes. It means accepting your mistakes while being kind and constructive rather than harsh. It's about focusing on what you can do better while being okay with making mistakes. This is important because it ensures your desire for change comes from love and a wish to do well rather than a fear of being judged.

As you practice self-compassion more, you will likely notice positive changes in your emotional and mental health. You may feel less stressed and anxious, find more inner peace, and improve your overall well-being. Developing self-compassion may take time, but its benefits are significant and lasting.

Set Personal Boundaries

Personal boundaries are essential for self-love and emotional safety. Clear boundaries help us decide how we want others to treat us, protect our personal values, and support our emotional health. When we create boundaries, we ensure that our needs are respected and show that we care about ourselves. Healthy boundaries help us keep our values intact. They allow us to express what is important to us and enable us to interact with others in ways that respect our dignity. For example, if honesty matters to you, a boundary requesting honest communication ensures that your interactions reflect your values. This way, you can avoid situations that might hurt your integrity or emotional well-being.

Types of Boundaries

Different types of boundaries play various protective roles in our lives. Physical boundaries define our personal space and physical safety. For example, a physical boundary could express your preferences about personal touch or how close someone can get to you. Emotional boundaries, on the other hand, guard our feelings and emotional well-being. They help us manage how much emotional energy we give and receive from others, which prevents us from becoming overwhelmed or emotionally drained. Mental boundaries are all about our thoughts, beliefs, and opinions. They protect our mental clarity and independence. Each type of boundary has a specific role in protecting our overall well-being.

Communicate Your Boundaries

Setting boundaries is one thing, but you must also communicate them to others. Boundaries should be communicated in a way that ensures they are understood and respected by others. Communicate your boundaries clearly; instead of hinting or assuming that others will understand your boundaries, it is important to articulate them explicitly.

Use "I" statements to explain your boundaries to other people. For example, saying, "I feel uncomfortable when..." or "I need some time alone after work to recharge" clearly communicates your boundary without blaming the other person. It's also important to explain how your boundary might link to your inner child. For instance, you might ask that the other person keep a calm tone during disagreements because you were exposed to screaming matches as a child.

This approach creates understanding and reduces the likelihood of defensive responses from the other person.

You can use the following steps to communicate your boundaries:

1. Be clear and straightforward. Being straightforward means avoiding ambiguity so the other person knows what you expect from them. If someone doesn't adhere to your boundary, kindly but firmly reiterate your point to reinforce its importance.

2. State your need directly. Explain your specific need in terms of what you'd like rather than what you don't want to help frame the request positively and constructively.

3. Accept any discomfort that arises. The initial awkwardness or guilt is often a sign of growth and change, especially if you've previously struggled with maintaining boundaries due to codependency or people-pleasing tendencies.

Examples of healthy boundaries include declining invitations to activities you are not interested in, expressing your feelings responsibly, talking about your experiences honestly, addressing problems directly with the person involved, and making your expectations clear rather than assuming people will figure them out. These kinds of requests uphold your boundaries and nurture healthy relationships based on mutual respect and understanding.

Adjustment Is Okay

You change over time, so it's only natural for your boundaries to evolve well. As you grow and change, your needs and limits can shift, so it's important to regularly reassess your boundaries and ensure they still serve your best interests. Reflecting on your experiences can help identify areas where you may need stronger boundaries or some kind of modification. For instance, a once-sufficient communication boundary might require reinforcement if someone else frequently challenges or overlooks it.

Major life changes such as starting a new job, entering a relationship, or experiencing a loss can also prompt a reevaluation of your boundaries. During these times, your priorities and capacities can change, which makes it essential to adapt your boundaries accordingly. Be flexible and open to adjusting your boundaries so you can work through new circumstances while prioritizing your emotional health.

Nourishing Activities for the Soul

Self-love happens when you take care of yourself, and that can mean adding fulfilling activities to daily life. You want to identify activities that resonate with your inner self. They should bring joy, relaxation, and satisfaction, nurturing you from within.

Add Joyful Activities to Your Day

Start by reflecting on past experiences where you felt really happy and content. What were you doing? Was it during a walk in nature, while painting, reading a book, or perhaps during a yoga session? These activities allow you to reconnect with parts of yourself that may have been neglected over time. For some, it might be creative activities like drawing or writing. Physical activities like dancing or hiking might bring the most joy to others. Whatever you choose, it needs to work for you.

Once you've identified these soul-nourishing activities, the next step is to craft a realistic plan to make them part of your daily life. It requires intention and mindfulness to ensure these practices become a regular part of your routine. Begin by setting achievable goals for your chosen activities. For example, if you enjoy painting, dedicate a specific time each week, even if it's just an hour, to immerse yourself in this activity. Similarly, if walking in nature brings you peace, schedule regular walks in your local park. The idea is to prioritize these activities without overwhelming yourself, so start small and gradually increase the frequency as they become habitual.

A balanced plan should also consider your current schedule. It may be necessary to make some adjustments to fit in these soul-nourishing activities. You might need to let go of certain non-essential tasks or delegate some of your responsibilities to free up time. It's important to remember that you are not trying to add more to your plate but rather making mindful choices that prioritize your well-being.

The Benefits of Nourishing Activities

Fulfilling activities have a profound impact on mental and emotional health. Participating in enjoyable and meaningful activities can reduce stress, anxiety, and depression while improving overall happiness and life satisfaction (Martinez, 2023). When you consistently do activities that bring you joy, your brain releases chemicals like endorphins and serotonin, which improve your mood and create a sense of well-being. Over time, these positive feelings contribute to improved mental health and act as a buffer against the negative effects of stress and adversity.

When you do activities that bring you joy, you also develop a deeper connection with yourself. This creates an opportunity to tune in to your needs, desires, and emotions, which increases self-awareness and emotional intelligence. As you strengthen this connection, you build a stronger foundation for self-love and acceptance. This process can heal old wounds from your childhood and help release pent-up emotions so that you have space for new, positive experiences.

A Supportive Community

A community of support is another vital part of adding fulfilling activities into your daily life. Connecting with others who share similar interests can provide motivation, encouragement, and a sense of belonging. Join clubs, groups, or online communities focused on activities you enjoy. It could be a book club, a local hiking group, or a crafting circle; regardless of your choice, these communities offer valuable opportunities to meet like-minded individuals and form meaningful relationships.

Being part of a supportive community can make your chosen activities more enjoyable and improve your emotional well-being. Social connections are known to improve mental health and provide a network of support during challenging times (Reblin & Uchino, 2018). Sharing your experiences, learning from others, and celebrating mutual achievements can be incredibly rewarding and reinforce your commitment to self-love practices.

Consider inviting friends or family members to join you in your activities or ask if you can accompany them in what they do. This shared experience can strengthen bonds and create lasting memories. Virtual communities or forums can be equally beneficial if you prefer solitude, as they offer a platform to connect with others while maintaining your personal space.

Daily Rituals for Self-Care

Self-love should be part of your everyday life, and that means establishing daily rituals that focus on self-care. These rituals—intentional actions carried out regularly—signify a commitment to looking after yourself both physically and emotionally. Frequently doing these activities can create a foundation of stability and self-appreciation.

Daily self-care rituals are deliberate actions that become touchstones throughout the day and reinforce your dedication to your health and happiness. These routines can range from simple activities such as morning stretches and evening relaxation techniques to more structured practices like meditation or journaling. The important thing is ensuring that these activities are meaningful and contribute positively to your sense of well-being.

Self-Care Examples

A great way to start the day with self-care is through mindfulness. You could take a few moments to do deep breathing exercises, set intentions for the day, or have a brief meditation session. Mindfulness helps to center your mind, reduce stress, and increase awareness, which provides a calming start to the day. Guided meditations or listening to calming music can also soothe the mind.

During the day, you can practice self-care by eating healthy, being mindful, and finding moments to pause between your hectic schedule. For example, you can take a walk during your lunch break or send a text message to a close friend. These activities allow you to get your work done while prioritizing your well-being and healing. Evening unwinding practices are equally important. They might include activities like reading a book, taking a calming bath, or doing a digital detox by avoiding screens for an hour before bed. These evening routines can help you unwind from the day's activities to restful sleep.

Personalize Your Self-Care Routine

Finding a personalized self-care routine that works for you takes some degree of experimentation. Everyone's needs and preferences vary, so you should try different activities until you find what works best. Start by considering your lifestyle and existing commitments. Ask yourself questions like:

- What time of day am I most stressed?

- When do I have pockets of free time?

- Do I prefer active or passive forms of relaxation?

From there, identify small, manageable activities that can fit into your daily schedule. For instance, if mornings are typically rushed, a quick five-minute meditation may be more feasible than an extended yoga session.

Starting simple is beneficial. Acknowledge what currently brings you joy and solace, and focus on doing those things. Experiment with various practices and pay close attention to what makes you feel good about yourself. Remember that self-care should never feel like an added burden but rather a supportive, enjoyable aspect of daily living. Still, approach this process with realistic expectations. Often, we fall into the trap of creating overly ambitious routines that are unsustainable in the long run. It's more sustainable to begin with small changes and gradually build upon them. If an elaborate morning routine seems daunting, start with one or two simple practices and progressively add more once they become habitual.

It's also helpful to establish certain non-negotiables within your self-care routine. These are the practices that are the most important to you and should be prioritized no matter the circumstances. For some, this might mean always making time for a morning run; for others, it could be ensuring they disconnect from work devices after a specific time each evening. Developing a sustainable self-care routine doesn't happen overnight. Begin small, perhaps incorporating one new practice every week or month. Gradually, these practices will add up and become a regular part of your daily life. Every habit you add can significantly impact your emotional well-being and healing your inner child.

Evaluate the Effects

It's also important to determine if your self-care rituals have the desired effect, which is an ongoing process. Regular self-care practices should improve your emotional awareness and make you more attuned to your feelings and reactions. Over time, these rituals create a loving relationship with yourself and serve as consistent reminders of your self-worth. Tracking moods, thoughts, and emotions through journaling can provide valuable insights into how these self-care practices impact your mental and emotional health. Pay attention to shifts in your mood, energy levels, and overall satisfaction with life. You may find a specific ritual works really well for you and decide to do it more often, but you could also discover that something else doesn't do much for your well-being, in which case you can replace it with another self-care activity.

Establishing and maintaining daily self-care rituals can provide immediate emotional relief and other benefits. Regular self-care has been shown to reduce symptoms of anxiety and depression, improve concentration, and increase overall happiness. Consistent self-care can lead to improved physical health and reduce risks related to heart disease, stroke, and other chronic conditions (Glowiak, 2024).

The ultimate goal of these daily self-care rituals is to cultivate a deeper connection with yourself, creating a loving relationship built on respect, care, and understanding. As you continue these practices, you'll likely notice an increased ability to tackle life's challenges with resilience and grace. You may also find yourself better equipped to support your loved ones and pursue your goals with renewed vigor. Just as the well-known advice on airplanes suggests putting on your own oxygen mask first before assisting others, prioritizing self-care allows you to show up fully for others. With a solid foundation of self-love, you are empowered to take on life's challenges with confidence and compassion.

Love Yourself

Various habits and practices can nurture self-love, which is essential to healing your inner child and achieving emotional freedom. Throughout this chapter, we've explored the powerful impact of positive affirmations, the importance of self-compassion over self-criticism, the necessity of setting personal boundaries, and the value of doing soul-nourishing activities. Each of these elements contributes to building a healthier relationship with yourself. Integrating these practices into your daily routine allows you to mend emotional wounds and develop a stronger sense of self-worth. These changes take time and patience. Healing from past trauma or emotional neglect is not a straightforward journey, but with consistent effort and self-kindness, you can make progress.

6

Healing Through Connection

Strong relationships can make a huge difference in soothing your inner wounds and nurturing the child within you who still yearns for care, compassion, and understanding. When you allow yourself to lean on others and accept support, you begin to break down the walls built out of past traumas and neglect. Solid connections allow you to heal and create space for growth, resilience, and newfound strength.

Building Supportive Networks

Knowing who to turn to during difficult times can help you feel less overwhelmed. Life's challenges can be scary, but having a reliable support network means you do not have to face them alone. Trusted friends and family can offer different perspectives, practical advice, or a listening ear. They can be there for you. This reassurance can ease the burden of hardships and make them seem more manageable. It also reinforces the idea that seeking help is not a sign of weakness; it's a step toward empowerment and resilience.

Identify Your Support Circle

Who can you rely on during difficult moments? It's important to recognize individuals who contribute positively to your emotional well-being, as they can help you feel less isolated. Often, these are people who listen without judgment, provide compassion, and offer consistent support.

Identifying your support circle is a critical step in your healing journey. Start by listing the people in your life who consistently show empathy, respect, and support. This might include friends, family members, or colleagues who show real interest in your feelings and experiences. Reflect on how each person affects your emotional state: Do they uplift you, or do they drain your energy? This exercise helps you discern which relationships are worth nurturing and which may need boundaries. Building a support circle begins with acknowledging and strengthening these connections with mutual respect and care.

Strong support systems provide a sense of belonging that helps you heal. The presence of supportive relationships reminds you that you are valued and accepted, regardless of your past experiences or current struggles. This sense of belonging decreases feelings of isolation and loneliness, which are common if you have faced emotional neglect or trauma. Surround yourself with people who care; you might have a renewed sense of hope and optimism that paves the way for emotional recovery.

Community Resources and Groups

Community activities offer opportunities to meet new people with similar interests and values. You could join a local club, volunteer for a cause you care about, or participate in neighborhood events to encounter interactions that create a sense of belonging. Community involvement combats loneliness and makes you feel accepted. They often serve as lifelines, especially if you feel you have no one else to turn to. Being part of a community gives you emotional support and encouragement, which are vital components of the healing process.

Support groups, specifically, are a way to broaden your network of supportive relationships. They bring together individuals who share similar experiences, creating a community filled with understanding and empathy. You can share stories, exchange advice, and offer mutual encouragement within these groups. The collective experience can validate your personal struggles and reduce feelings of isolation. Knowing that others have faced and overcome similar challenges can be empowering and give you the strength to keep going.

Your support networks can also offer alternative perspectives on your experiences. Sometimes, we are so deeply entrenched in our own emotions and thoughts that we struggle to see beyond our immediate pain. Supportive relationships provide fresh viewpoints that can show us new ways of thinking and problem-solving. These alternative perspectives broaden our understanding of the situation and inspire innovative approaches to healing and self-care.

Trust in Friendships

Trust allows us to be vulnerable without fear of judgment, something that is essential for healing. Trust is developed over time through repeated experiences showing reliability and safety within relationships. When trust is established, it gives us a secure environment where we can express our emotions openly and honestly. This vulnerability can help us address past wounds and increase personal growth. Through trusting relationships, we realize that we are not alone in our struggles, which can feel like the weight of our emotional burdens become lighter.

Building trust within a support network requires ongoing effort and openness. It doesn't just happen; trust requires a steady stream of positive interactions with others and a willingness to be vulnerable. You can deepen the connection and reinforce trust with others by sharing your thoughts and feelings and listening to them. Both of you should respect each other's boundaries and keep private information confidential. A solid foundation of trust ensures that the support network remains a safe space for all involved.

Professional Help

Healing from trauma is a complex process. While friends and family can provide significant emotional support, professionals offer specialized knowledge and skills. Therapists, counselors, and coaches play an instrumental role in the healing journey, offering expert insights and strategies suited to your specific challenges. They can help you uncover underlying issues, guide self-reflection, and develop personalized coping strategies. They also provide a neutral, non-judgmental space to discuss sensitive topics that might be difficult to talk about with loved ones. Their expertise can accelerate the healing process, making it more comprehensive and enduring.

Professionals have the training to help you manage complex emotions and will suggest tools and techniques to help you deal with stress, anxiety, and other symptoms of trauma. Professionals understand the importance of inner child work and can assist you with reparenting, self-compassion, and other techniques. They also ensure that you are supported in a structured and safe way so you can heal effectively in the long run.

The Importance of Vulnerability

Vulnerability should be found in any relationship where we want to build stronger connections and better healing experiences. Vulnerability opens us up to authentic interactions, which creates a relationship built on trust and honesty. Authenticity is about presenting our true selves without masks or defenses. We can communicate more openly when we show our vulnerabilities, leading to stronger connections. For instance, admitting fears, anxieties, or past traumas helps others understand you better and encourages empathy. This mutual understanding strengthens the relationship and provides a secure environment where both of you feel safe to express yourself freely.

The courage to be vulnerable means you are willing to take small risks gradually. Small doses of vulnerability help build your resilience and confidence over time. For instance, start telling someone a little bit about your day-to-day feelings; over time, it becomes easier to share more significant parts of your life. By taking these small steps, you can slowly break down the defensive walls built around your emotions and make room for real connections.

Vulnerability also allows you to resolve conflict through open communication. When you are willing to express your fears and concerns honestly, it becomes easier to talk about misunderstandings and disagreements. Vulnerability encourages both you and the other person to voice your perspectives without fear of judgment. It enables mutual understanding and reconciliation. For example, a couple who shares their vulnerabilities during an argument can better understand each other's viewpoints, which leads to healthier resolutions and a stronger bond.

Share Your Story

Sharing your personal experiences can lead to healing conversations and support from others. Talking about challenges or past hurts with your friends, family, or therapy groups is essential because these conversations can make you feel understood and less alone. For example, someone with anxiety might feel relief when they see they are not the only one struggling. This shared understanding can help everyone involved heal together as they learn from each other.

You also grow emotionally by being open about your struggles. When you share your weaknesses, you develop empathy and compassion for yourself and others. This growth helps you understand and respond to other people's needs better. For instance, sharing your personal story about childhood trauma can help you feel more empathy towards others dealing with the same situation and strengthen emotional connections.

However, it's important to set personal limits to stay safe while being open. Boundaries ensure that you share in a way that doesn't overwhelm you. Clearly stating what topics you are okay discussing helps create a safe space for sharing with others. For example, telling a friend that specific topics are off-limits respects your personal space while still allowing for honest conversations. But that also means you need to ask them about their boundaries. This helps create a supportive environment for healthy growth and connections.

Practice Self-Acceptance

Accepting yourself is another part of being brave enough to be open with others. Self-acceptance means understanding and accepting all parts of who you are, including your flaws and past mistakes. This helps you be kinder to yourself and can soften the inner voice that may hold you back. When you accept yourself, you become more willing to show your true self to others, which helps create closer relationships. For instance, recognizing your fears about being left alone can lead to honest talks about the fear of abandonment with your partner, helping them to understand you better.

Mindfulness can also help you become more open and vulnerable because it teaches you to focus on the present and notice your thoughts and feelings without judging them. This kind of awareness helps you deal with vulnerability in a balanced way and allows you to recognize your fears and insecurities without being overwhelmed. It makes it easier to handle vulnerability with a sense of calm and clarity, which, in turn, allows you to take emotional risks comfortably.

When we are open and show our true selves, we make it easier for others to do the same. This openness lets us build genuine connections and strong relationships. Being vulnerable is a sign of strength, not weakness. It takes bravery to face our fears, tell our truths, and be open to connecting and growing with others. Through being vulnerable, we start to heal emotionally, learn about ourselves, and grow as individuals.

Effective Communication Skills

Communication is a fundamental part of healthy relationships and emotional healing. But if you have experienced trauma or emotional neglect, especially as a child, then you may struggle to communicate well. However, you can still learn to communicate effectively, and that can open the door to deeper connections and self-discovery.

Assertiveness

Let's talk about assertiveness, which is a characteristic of good communication. Being assertive allows you to express your needs clearly without being aggressive or passive. This kind of communication respects both people's feelings and encourages mutual respect. For example, saying, "I feel overwhelmed and need some alone time," is better than getting angry or staying quiet. It helps you share your needs without causing conflict. Practicing assertive communication regularly creates an environment where everyone feels listened to and respected, enabling healthy emotional exchanges.

In practical terms, being assertive means practicing clear and direct statements about your needs and feelings. For example, using "I" statements such as "I need" or "I feel" instead of accusatory "you" statements goes a long way in reducing defensiveness and increasing understanding. In some cases, you can rehearse your assertive statements by practicing them in front of a mirror, especially if you struggle to speak up. Assertiveness training might be part of your therapy, or you could attend workshops on it, which can provide you with the skills needed to express yourself better.

Nonverbal Communication

Nonverbal cues—also known as body language—are a critical part of communication. In many cases, they convey emotions and intentions more powerfully than words. A comforting touch, sincere eye contact, or a relaxed posture can speak volumes about your feelings and engagement in a conversation. These nonverbal signals often align closely with our true emotions, which makes them essential tools for authentic communication. Being mindful of our own nonverbal signals and those of others can improve our understanding and empathy, creating a supportive and nurturing environment that is ideal for emotional healing.

As a child, you may have adopted some nonverbal cues that you still use today. For example, hunching your shoulders or looking down when someone is upset with you. It can help to become more attuned to both your own body language and that of others so you convey what you really mean. Techniques like maintaining comfortable eye contact, adopting an open and relaxed posture, and being mindful of facial expressions can significantly improve the quality of your interactions. Observing these cues allows for a deeper emotional connection and better empathic responses, making the relationship more nurturing.

Safe Spaces for Dialogue

Environments where open sharing is encouraged can lead to deeper and more meaningful connections. Safe spaces should make people feel welcome to express their thoughts and emotions without fear of judgment so they can develop trust and intimacy. This is particularly important as you heal from past traumas, as it provides a sanctuary where vulnerability is met with compassion. Simple practices like regular, uninterrupted conversations and active listening (where you give full attention to the speaker) can make a huge difference. Openness strengthens relationships and facilitates a more profound emotional release, which can be cathartic on your healing journey.

To create environments where sharing is welcomed, you should set aside dedicated time for meaningful conversations. Additionally, strategies like a no-interruption rule during discussions and creating rituals that improve connection can be helpful. For instance, you can schedule family meetings or regular check-ins with friends to develop a norm of openness and support within the relationship.

Feedback and Reflection

Another crucial part of communication in relationships is giving and getting helpful feedback. Helpful feedback is clear, practical, and meant to encourage growth instead of criticism. You should be open to receiving and providing feedback. To give feedback effectively, you should share your thoughts without blaming anyone and suggest improvements in a positive way. For example, instead of saying, "You never listen to me," you might say, "I feel ignored when I'm interrupted; could we wait until each person finishes speaking?" It's also crucial to accept feedback without getting defensive. Keep an open mind when someone gives you feedback, and be ready to see criticism as an opportunity to grow. Learning to do this helps with personal growth and strengthens relationships.

The skill of giving and receiving helpful feedback takes time to build. Workshops, books, and advice from mental health professionals can provide useful tips on how to give and accept feedback respectfully. Practicing this skill in safe settings where friends or partners can exchange feedback respectfully may be useful. If you are brave enough, ask someone for their input and be open to hearing them fully. In the end, communication involves more than just talking. It's about building a mix of spoken and unspoken interactions that increase understanding, respect, and emotional safety.

Empathy and Active Listening

Active listening and empathy, known as empathetic listening, can greatly improve relationships. This type of listening includes both spoken and body language that shows you truly care about someone's feelings. These skills help people feel heard and supported, which makes them more willing to share and have meaningful discussions. For someone recovering from trauma or emotional neglect, this kind of connection can be very healing.

Empathy

Empathy is essential for building strong relationships and helping people heal. When people understand each other's feelings, they validate one another, and this shared understanding is key to supportive relationships. Empathy allows you to feel what another person is going through. It helps them know that their feelings matter and that they are not alone in their path to recovery, just like you aren't alone in yours.

Empathetic listening requires us to reflect back on the emotions we hear from others. Phrases like "You sound really frustrated" or "It seems like you're feeling overwhelmed" demonstrate that you are attuned to the other person's emotional state. These kinds of words are something you can look for in your relationships to determine if other people also empathize with you. If they do, you may feel that they validate your feelings and encourage you to talk more about your emotions, which allows for greater self-awareness and emotional clarity. Empathetic listening requires setting aside your biases and ego to genuinely understand another's perspective.

Active Listening

Active listening is critical because it makes people feel heard and valued. Unlike just hearing someone talk, active listening requires your full attention and awareness of what is said and how it's said. This means keeping eye contact, nodding, and responding with words to show you are paying attention so that the other person can share openly, knowing their words matter. Active listening is about understanding what the other person is trying to say and showing that you get it. It means understanding the emotions and messages behind their words.

Active listening should happen in your day-to-day conversations and specifically during therapy. The counselor listens to you, and you should listen to the counselor and yourself. This type of listening can help in everyday relationships as it improves understanding and creates strong connections. Overall, active listening is a technique that involves paying close attention and asking questions to really understand the emotions behind what someone is saying.

Using this technique in personal relationships can change how you relate to and support each other.

An accepting attitude is also necessary for active listening. We need to respect each other's rights to think and feel differently without passing judgment. Respect in active listening means viewing people as individuals with their own experiences and recognizing that they can grow at their own speed. This acceptance helps build deep, meaningful connections where we feel safe sharing our thoughts and feelings without fear of being judged or ignored.

It is essential to recognize what empathy and active listening are not. Commanding, warning, lecturing, judging, blaming, shaming, analyzing, probing, humoring, and distracting are all barriers to effective listening. These behaviors shut down self-exploration and conversation. Instead, it creates a relationship where neither of you can communicate well. The focus should be on an atmosphere of mutual respect and collaboration, allowing for an authentic and trusting connection.

Respond With Compassion

It's possible to establish emotional safety by communicating with understanding and support, both to yourself and in response to other people's emotions. Responding with empathy and without judgment creates a safe space for open and honest communication. For instance, if someone shares a painful experience, a response like, "That must have been really tough for you," shows empathy and validates their feelings. This acknowledgment helps build trust and encourages further sharing, which reinforces the emotional bond. Expressions of support like, "I am here for you" or "You don't have to go through this alone," can increase a person's sense of security and belonging. You want to identify relationships where you get compassionate responses because those are the people who will listen to and support you.

Keep Triggers in Mind

Triggers are specific words, actions, or situations that can evoke intense emotional responses based on past experiences. They can come up easily in conversation, so you need to be aware of these triggers to help manage conversations more mindfully. Think of triggers both for yourself and the other person. For example, if you know that discussing certain topics makes your partner anxious, you can approach those subjects with extra care and sensitivity. This awareness prevents unnecessary harm and creates healthier interactions. By recognizing your own triggers, you can better communicate your needs and boundaries so you can have healthier conversations that support your emotional well-being.

Dealing With Triggering Relationships

Some relationships can trigger your emotional wounds, but they are still important in the healing process. You will need to recognize specific individuals or behaviors that bring up negative emotions. You gain the power to address them head-on when you identify these triggers. For example, if interactions with your parents consistently lead to feelings of inadequacy or anger, acknowledge this pattern so that you can start taking the necessary actions to decrease their effect on you. This self-awareness enables you to manage your emotional responses proactively, which may lead to better mental health.

Negative behavior often results from unresolved emotional issues, and some actions can worsen emotional pain. By paying attention to situations that cause emotional distress, you can learn to expect triggers and respond better. For example, if birthdays always make you feel sad about your childhood, recognizing this can help you prepare mentally and emotionally for future celebrations and decrease your emotional response.

Establish Healthy Boundaries

Once again, boundaries are vital to maintaining healthy relationships and protecting your emotional well-being. Boundaries help prevent conversations and actions that might otherwise hinder your healing. Clear boundaries ensure that your personal needs and limits are respected, which reduces the potential for emotional harm. For instance, you might limit conversations about certain topics with specific individuals who are prone to causing you distress. This kind of intentional boundary-setting can create a safer emotional environment and enable more productive and positive interactions.

Setting boundaries is about creating conditions conducive to healing. Therapeutic boundaries may involve physical space, such as spending less time with triggering individuals, or emotional limits, like refraining from discussing sensitive subjects. Stick to these boundaries to prevent old wounds from being reopened so that you can focus on positive conversations that help you heal. Communicate these boundaries respectfully to others and respect their boundaries in return.

Get Professional Help

In difficult relationships, getting help from experts is very important. Therapists use different methods to help you deal with your emotions and challenging relationships. Therapists, counselors, and mental health professionals can teach you how to challenge unhelpful thoughts and replace them with more balanced ones. It can help change how they feel about certain situations. These professionals also create a safe space to talk about your feelings, understand where you come from, and help you build healthier relationships. Trust is essential in therapy; it enables you to face your relationship issues and work towards positive changes.

They often use mindfulness and techniques to help you control your emotions. Mindfulness helps you stay focused on the present, which can help you handle your emotional triggers with a calmer mindset. Techniques for managing emotions, like deep breathing and mental imagery, help control strong feelings so they don't interfere with your daily life.

Therapists can also help you understand and fix power issues in your relationships. When one person has more power, it can make your emotional pain worse and make healing harder. Professional help allows you to address these power issues, encourages fairness and shared decisions, and helps you set boundaries. Talking about power dynamics helps resolve conflicts and leads to healthier ways of interacting with others.

Choose Empowering Interactions

Emotional growth happens when you have relationships that validate your emotions and minimize your triggers. Validation from supportive individuals can bring you comfort and reinforce the progress you have made in healing. Look for connections with individuals who understand and respect your healing process. These relationships should have open communication, active listening, and empathy, creating an environment where you feel heard and valued. It should be based on a mutual understanding that nurtures emotional safety and a sense of security.

Social support from friends and family members who validate your experiences and emotions can help a lot. Share your experiences with trusted individuals to get validation and different perspectives, and it will reduce feelings of loneliness while improving your emotional resilience. Trusted friends and family members offer comfort and reassurance during challenging times, and there will be plenty of those moments as you heal your inner child.

Support groups can also provide a platform for sharing, listening, and understanding as people share similar experiences. The individuals in your group may even become some of your closest and most trusted relationships. Participating in community activities or support groups combats loneliness and gives you a sense of belonging. These connections become a buffer against emotional stress and positively impact your well-being.

Make a Connection

Relationships play an important part in healing emotional wounds, and we need to remember the powerful impact that supportive connections can have on our journey toward self-discovery and growth. Individuals who truly listen and offer compassion can create a network of support that helps us reconnect with our inner child. Whether it's through community involvement, professional guidance, or forging closer ties with family and friends, these connections provide the safety and trust necessary for true healing.

Be vulnerable within these relationships and share your true self so you can develop authentic relationships based on mutual understanding. This will strengthen your existing connections and offer new perspectives and approaches to our emotional struggles. Healing happens gradually and requires patience, but leaning into these supportive networks empowers you to face your challenges with resilience and hope.

7

Therapeutic Techniques for Healing

Healing your inner child may require various therapeutic techniques that focus on your emotional well-being. These methods can help you address your past trauma, and many of them offer practical approaches to healing and building self-compassion. By exploring these techniques, you can develop strategies to reconnect with your younger self, as they provide the care and understanding you may have missed as a child.

Inner Child Therapy Concepts

Inner child therapy, while focused on dealing with past traumas, is based on the goal of creating a better present and future. We may still have emotional needs from childhood, so nurturing them can help us grow and become more resilient. This method recognizes that many adult issues stem from unresolved childhood experiences, and through nurturing these needs, we can initiate a healing process. As adults, we have the power to rewrite the stories we learned as children in an attempt to develop a healthier, more compassionate relationship with ourselves.

Reparenting

A big part of inner child therapy is reparenting, a technique where you provide yourself with the nurturing and support you may have lacked during your childhood. Reparenting requires speaking kindly to yourself, setting healthy boundaries, and creating a safe internal environment. For instance, if someone experienced neglect or harsh criticism as a child, they might practice affirmations like, "I am deserving of love and care," to counteract those negative messages. If you consistently offer yourself compassion and understanding, you begin to heal old wounds and develop a healthier perception of yourself.

It may help to have some guidelines for reparenting techniques. Start by identifying specific unmet needs from your childhood. Reflect on what you lacked emotionally: Is it affection, validation, or safety? Once identified, consciously work on fulfilling those needs in your current life. For instance, if you didn't get recognition for good work as a child, you may want to pat yourself on the back when you achieve something in your typical day. Create a routine where you check in with yourself daily, offering positive reinforcement and comfort. Over time, this practice will help build a supportive internal dialogue that encourages healing.

Visualization

Visualization techniques are another part of inner child therapy and help you reconnect with your inner child to facilitate healing through practical and imaginative methods. A common visualization technique is closing your eyes and picturing your younger self in a safe, comforting place. You can have a loving conversation with this inner child, which allows for the expression of buried emotions and fears. These visualizations can be tremendously helpful to build self-compassion and release pent-up feelings.

Here is an exercise you can try right now:

1. Begin by finding a quiet place free from distractions.

2. Close your eyes and take deep breaths to center yourself.

3. Visualize your inner child: How do they look? What are they feeling?

4. Talk to them and ask what they need.

5. Give them reassurance that everything will be okay.

Integrating the Inner Child

Bringing fun and joyful experiences into adult life is essential for healing and self-care. We often ignore playfulness as adults, but it is necessary to stay emotionally healthy. Activities that gave you joy as a child–like drawing, playing music, or being outdoors–can bring back feelings of wonder and creativity. These activities remind us that making time for enjoyment is necessary because it is crucial for our emotional health.

To keep joyful experiences a regular part of your life, start by making them a priority. Set aside specific times each week for activities that make you happy. Make a list of your childhood favorites, and try to do at least one activity every few days, even if it's just for a few minutes. It could be dancing, painting, or reading a favorite book–whatever you choose, these activities help you balance your responsibilities with your emotional well-being.

Role of Cognitive Behavioral Therapy (CBT)

CBT provides a safe place for you to look at your past trauma and how it affects your current thoughts and actions. CBT helps address negative thinking that often comes from unresolved childhood trauma. It requires that you look at irrational beliefs that started in your childhood and work to change them into positive and realistic thoughts. With CBT, you can begin to recognize and change harmful thoughts, leading to healing and better emotional health.

It often includes activities like writing about your trauma, telling a therapist about it, or acting out situations. These activities help you face and deal with painful memories in a safe way, which can lessen your emotional load. Confronting these memories can change how you understand and react to past events, reducing their negative effects.

CBT is practical and can be used in real life. The techniques learned in therapy can be applied in everyday situations, making CBT useful and easy to access. For example, you might practice changing negative thoughts during a tough work meeting or use relaxation methods before a difficult conversation. Using these skills in daily life can help you find long-term healing outside of your therapy sessions.

Another helpful part of CBT is that it can be changed to fit your needs. Therapists can adjust CBT methods to match your specific problems and strengths to ensure that the therapy is personal and effective. CBT can be modified to deal with the unique ways negative thoughts show up during anxiety, depression, or PTSD. This personalization makes the treatment more effective, giving you support that directly addresses your challenges.

Identify Negative Thoughts

CBT focuses on identifying and challenging unhelpful beliefs and thought patterns formed from childhood experiences. These negative beliefs can include feeling unworthy, guilty, or overly critical of yourself. For example, a child who feels ignored might believe they are unlovable. In CBT, these thoughts are examined closely. The therapist helps the person question these beliefs by asking questions like, "What proof do you have for this belief?" or "Can you see this situation in another way?" Through this process, you can begin to view your thoughts differently and reduce the power of negative patterns.

Cognitive Restructuring

Cognitive restructuring, which helps you change negative thoughts and develop a positive mindset, is part of CBT. With this process, you spot harmful thinking patterns—like thinking everything is bad or expecting the worst—and replace them with more realistic thoughts. For instance, someone who thinks "bad things always happen to me" can learn to see this as an exaggerated way of thinking. Cognitive restructuring can change this thought to something more reasonable, such as "Although bad things have happened, good things also happen, and I am strong enough to face challenges." This change reduces negative effects and builds resilience and confidence.

Emotional Regulation

CBT is essential for managing feelings during stressful times. Childhood trauma can make it hard to regulate emotions and cause strong and unmanageable reactions in adults. CBT provides techniques like mindfulness exercises and deep breathing to help you stay calm and handle your emotions. If you use these methods frequently, you can gain better control over how you respond emotionally and avoid being overwhelmed by stress. Take a moment to breathe and respond thoughtfully instead of reacting quickly; it will significantly improve your emotional well-being.

Goals and Progress Tracking

Goal setting and tracking progress in CBT are important for healing because setting clear, realistic goals gives direction and purpose. For example, you might want to challenge one negative thought each week. As you use CBT, you need to track your progress to keep you accountable and help you celebrate small wins. Keeping a daily journal of achievements lets you see your growth and stay motivated. These recorded successes support positive changes and motivate your ongoing efforts for better mental health.

For those who have experienced childhood trauma, CBT can be demanding but rewarding. It involves facing deep beliefs and feelings, which may be uncomfortable. However, the benefits include better self-awareness, emotional control, and changing unhelpful thoughts. As you work through CBT, you may develop healthier relationships, improved self-esteem, and greater life satisfaction.

Mental health professionals understand CBT and can guide you through a structured healing process, offering proven tools and techniques. This understanding helps them provide you with strong support so you can overcome past trauma and create a healthier future.

Art and Creative Therapies

Art and creative therapies can be a great way to heal, express your feelings, and understand your experiences. Creative activities allow you to show complex emotions without words, which makes it easier to deal with feelings that are hard to express. Activities like painting, sculpting, or drawing can bring out hidden feelings and turn them into something visible. This process can lighten your emotional struggles and give you a sense of relief and release. Using art therapies with traditional methods, like cognitive-behavioral therapy or talk therapy, can provide a complete healing experience. The insights from creative activities can improve your thinking and emotional skills learned in these therapies, offering a well-rounded approach to healing.

Therapeutic Benefits of Creativity

Art therapy sessions use activities that help you express your emotions. Techniques such as drawing or sculpting with clay can release hidden feelings and provide a new understanding of your inner world. Materials like clay can help you shape your emotions into real forms. This can be especially helpful if you struggle to express yourself verbally, giving you a different way to understand and release your feelings.

Doing art activates the brain's reward system, which is important for reducing anxiety and increasing happiness. When you create, your brain releases dopamine, a chemical that makes you feel good (Nash, 2018). For example, finishing a piece of art can lead to feelings of accomplishment and joy, which helps to overcome fear or sadness. This positive effect on mental health emphasizes the healing power of creativity.

Creative therapy is effective at helping you become stronger mentally. If you participate in art activities frequently, you learn how to deal with stress and tough times. Repetitive activities like knitting or woodworking can calm the mind, much like meditation. These hobbies keep you focused and help take your mind off negative thoughts, leading to relaxation and clear thinking. The benefits of creative therapy increase when done regularly. Making creative activities a habit can help with your emotional growth and self-discovery, so stick to these routines to boost the positive impact and experience better overall well-being and mental strength.

Mindfulness in Art

Being mindful during art amplifies the healing experience by encouraging you to focus on your present emotions without judgment. Creating art mindfully invites you to immerse yourself in the process, paying attention to sensations, thoughts, and feelings as they arise. It increases your self-awareness and acceptance, which helps you confront your emotions in a safe space. For example, mindful painting can help you explore feelings of anger or grief by observing the movement of your brushstrokes and the colors you choose. It helps create a deeper understanding of your emotions.

Consider adding mindfulness practices into your creative sessions to fully benefit from creative therapies. Focus on the sensory experiences involved in the creative process, such as the texture of materials or the rhythm of movements. This intentional awareness can increase the emotional impact and contribute to your overall well-being.

Community and Connection

Group art projects build a sense of community and help emotional growth. Working on art together creates a supportive space where you feel connected and understood. These activities strengthen friendships and create a support network, which is essential as you recover from trauma. For example, working on a mural together can encourage people to share their stories and listen to others, promoting understanding and respect.

Benefits of Guided Imagery

Guided imagery is a useful technique that helps you relax and heal emotional pain by creating clear mental images. This method uses our natural ability to imagine, allowing us to picture calming and comforting scenes. Guided imagery can help you connect with your inner child, address past hurts, and improve your emotional health.

Emotional Safe Space

Guided imagery can help create safe emotional spaces. These are places in your mind where you can feel comfort and calm during stress or emotional challenges. Imagine closing your eyes and picturing a peaceful beach with gentle waves or a warm cabin in a quiet forest. The clearer and more vivid the image, the better it helps you feel safe and relaxed. In these spaces, your mind can unwind, which may decrease the physical and mental effects of anxiety and trauma.

To create these emotionally safe spaces, you need practice and patience. It helps to be in a quiet place without distractions like TVs or phones. Soft, calming music can improve the experience by hiding background noise and encouraging relaxation. Before starting the visualization, trying a relaxation technique, like deep breathing or tensing and relaxing your muscles, is helpful. This gets your body and mind ready for a deeper, more impactful experience.

Heal Past Wounds

Visualization exercises focused on childhood memories can be life-changing. These exercises let you revisit critical moments from your past in a safe way. For instance, someone might picture themselves as a child during a tough time but change the scene to include caring people or protective elements that were missing back then. This act of rethinking past events helps you recognize and let go of feelings tied to those memories. Facing these memories directly enables you to start to heal emotional scars that have affected your well-being for a long time.

Personal guides can be helpful during visualization exercises. These guides can be people, animals, or spiritual figures that provide support and comfort during the visualization. They help you deal with challenging memories and offer the reassurance needed to face and process these experiences. Over time, these guides can become important companions in your emotional journey as they provide steady support and advice.

Use Positive Anchors

Visualizing positive experiences is an integral part of guided imagery. This technique helps strengthen good feelings and beliefs about ourselves. For example, by regularly imagining good outcomes and positive scenarios, our brains form new pathways (Miles, n.d.). These pathways support actions and thoughts that boost self-esteem and create a more positive view of life. Using visualization frequently makes it easier to feel these positive emotions when times are tough. In practice, this could mean visualizing reaching personal goals or handling stressful situations well. Athletes often use similar methods to enhance their performance by imagining successful results. These positive visualizations help the brain act as if these successes have already happened, which increases confidence and motivation.

How to Use Guided Imagery

To get started with guided imagery, consider using scripts or recordings. These resources provide structured guidance and make it easier for beginners and experienced individuals to engage with the process effectively. As your familiarity with guided imagery grows, you can personalize these scripts based on your specific interests and needs to deepen the experience. Experiment with different scenarios and techniques to help discover what resonates most with you and heal your inner child.

Visualization sessions should ideally be a regular part of your routine to maximize the benefits. Consistent practice, several times a week over a period of months, improves the effectiveness of guided imagery. Daily practice may be beneficial if you are dealing with particular issues or illnesses. Over time, this regular engagement helps develop healthier coping mechanisms and supports your journey toward emotional healing.

Mindfulness techniques can also be used with guided imagery. Practices like mindful breathing or body scanning before starting a guided imagery session can increase relaxation and focus. By being present in the moment and attuned to your body's sensations, you can more effectively immerse yourself in your visualizations and amplify the healing potential.

Guided imagery nurtures a deep connection with the inner child, helping you understand and meet your emotional needs that may have been neglected in the past. It provides a space for your inner child to be heard and healed, which creates greater self-compassion and emotional resilience. This, in turn, supports your mental health and well-being for a more fulfilling life.

Somatic Experiencing and Body Awareness

Another popular method for healing trauma is somatic therapy, which focuses on the link between the mind and body to show how physical feelings can affect emotions. Somatic experiencing, a type of somatic therapy created by Dr. Peter Levine, helps people process trauma by improving body awareness and dealing with physical feelings related to their emotions.

Somatic experiencing is based on the idea that trauma affects both the mind and the body. When people experience trauma, their bodies often hold onto the physical reactions connected to those events. These reactions can show up as tension, pain, or other physical issues even after the trauma has occurred. Somatic experiencing helps people understand and work through these physical signs of trauma by paying attention to their bodily sensations.

Body-based therapies can be helpful for recovering from trauma. Trauma can impair thinking skills and make traditional cognitive-behavioral therapies less effective. Additionally, exposure therapy, often used in cognitive-behavioral treatment, can lead to many people quitting because it feels too confrontational. As a result, using body-oriented methods alongside these treatments has become more popular in the last 10 years (Kuhfuß et al., 2021).

Somatic experiencing has become known as a helpful treatment for PTSD, as it helps clients focus on their internal feelings and sensations. The idea is to change how trauma affects their stress responses and to assist people in finishing the physical and emotional reactions they experienced during the trauma, helping them resolve ongoing stress and emotional problems.

Tune Into Sensations

The somatic process begins with developing body awareness. A therapist will guide you in paying attention to your internal sensations, such as tightness in the chest or a knot in the stomach. This awareness brings hidden emotions linked to your childhood trauma to the surface. For example, an individual might realize that their chronic back pain is connected to feelings of fear or helplessness experienced during a traumatic childhood event. Recognizing these connections is the first step toward achieving emotional release and healing.

Your therapist will encourage you to take moments throughout your day to check in with your body. Simple exercises like closing the eyes, taking deep breaths, and scanning the body from head to toe can reveal areas of tension or discomfort. It's important to notice these sensations without judgment to help you become more attuned to your physical and emotional states. This practice can greatly help you to identify and process hidden emotions.

Grounding Techniques

Grounding techniques are another vital aspect of somatic therapies. Grounding reconnects you with your present moment and body to create a sense of safety and stability. Trauma can often leave us feeling disconnected from ourselves and our surroundings, which results in a constant state of anxiety or hypervigilance. Grounding exercises help mitigate these effects by anchoring us in the "here and now." For instance, grounding can involve practices like feeling one's feet firmly planted on the ground, holding onto a tangible object like a smooth stone, or doing deep, mindful breathing. These exercises draw attention away from distressing thoughts and back to your body's immediate experience. As a result, they can reduce anxiety and create a sense of calm and control.

Another effective grounding technique is the "4-7-8" breathing exercise. With this technique, you inhale for four seconds, hold your breath for seven seconds, and then exhale slowly for eight seconds. This controlled breathing pattern activates the parasympathetic nervous system, which counters your body's stress response, leading to a calming effect. You can practice these techniques regularly to improve your ability to remain grounded and stable, even when faced with stressors reminding you of past traumas.

Integrate Body and Mind

Integrating body-centered practices like yoga or mindful walking also contributes to emotional awareness and healing. Yoga, for example, combines physical poses, breath control, and meditation. It encourages you to connect deeply with your body and creates awareness of how you hold tension and emotion physically. Through regular practice, yoga can help you release stored trauma from your body, which gives you a sense of relief and well-being.

Mindful walking is another possibility and requires paying close attention to each step taken, the movement of muscles, and the sensation of the ground beneath your feet. This practice has physical benefits and amplifies mindfulness, allowing you to stay present and connected with your body. Walking in nature can increase these effects and offer additional restorative benefits that support peace and relaxation.

In practice, therapists using somatic experiencing may guide you through a combination of exercises that involve tracking physical sensations and releasing built-up energy. You allow your body to process these reactions gradually and safely, which helps to achieve a state of equilibrium and resilience. This approach, rooted in understanding the body's role in storing and expressing trauma, creates a different way of healing that traditional talk therapies may overlook.

Try Different Healing Therapies

Various therapeutic methods can help you heal your inner child. Techniques like reparenting, visualization, and integrating playful experiences into daily life can help you begin to address unresolved childhood traumas. These methods focus on self-compassion and encourage the development of healthier emotional habits to create a nurturing environment within oneself. Reconnecting with your younger self through these practices initiates an impactful healing process that deals with past hurts and sets the stage for a more balanced and fulfilling adult life. These therapeutic activities help rebuild self-esteem, establish safe internal spaces, and embrace joy. As you explore and apply these techniques, you empower yourself to rewrite old narratives and develop a compassionate relationship with your inner child.

8

Practical Tools for
Daily Healing

Meditation and deep breathing exercises are compelling avenues for healing, inviting you to become more present with your thoughts, emotions, and physical sensations. You can center yourself through mindfulness practices if you open a nurturing space for emotional well-being and self-awareness. This chapter explores how integrating these practices into daily life can ease emotional distress and provide a pathway to connect with your inner child.

Meditation and Deep Breathing Exercises

Healing is a process that requires patience and consistent effort. Mindfulness—a practice that helps you become more aware of your thoughts, emotions, and physical sensations—

can help you process trauma. It provides a comfortable way to soothe emotional distress and increase self-awareness.

Understanding Meditation

Meditation is a cornerstone of mindfulness practices. It involves focusing attention and eliminating the stream of jumbled thoughts that may be crowding your mind. This focus can lead to better emotional regulation and a deep sense of inner peace. Meditation encourages us to connect with our inner child, which is necessary to recover from trauma and emotional neglect. Through this connection, you can begin to heal old wounds and improve your emotional well-being.

There are various styles of meditation, each catering to different preferences and needs. One common style is guided meditation, where an instructor leads the meditator through specific visualizations and instructions. It is particularly useful for beginners who might feel lost or distracted when meditating alone. Guided meditation provides a structured framework that makes it easier to maintain focus and achieve a deeper state of relaxation.

Another form of meditation is body scan meditation, which involves mentally scanning the body from head to toe and taking note of any sensations of tension or discomfort. This heightens awareness of bodily sensations and emotional states. It allows you to release pent-up stress and develop a compassionate relationship with your body, contributing to overall emotional balance.

Sitting meditation is another popular style. In this practice, you sit comfortably with a straight back, either on the floor or in a chair, and focus on your breathing. The simplicity of sitting meditation makes it accessible and easy to add to daily routines. It's a versatile method that can be practiced almost anywhere and anytime, making it a useful tool to manage stress and improve self-awareness throughout the day.

Walking meditation is yet another ideal option if you find sitting still challenging. You should walk slowly and mindfully while paying close attention to each step and the sensations in your feet and legs. Walking meditation combines the benefits of movement with mindfulness, which makes it a great option if you feel restless or anxious during traditional meditation.

Benefits of Deep Breathing

Breathing exercises are part of many mindfulness practices, serving as a way to calm the mind and body. Simple breathing techniques can be incredibly effective to soothe emotional distress. Here are a few deep breathing exercises to try.

- **Deep Belly Breathing**: Inhale deeply through the nose, allowing your abdomen to expand. Exhale slowly through the mouth. This type of breathing activates the body's relaxation response and helps to reduce anxiety and tension.

- **Box Breathing**: Inhale for a count of four, hold the breath for a count of four, exhale for a count of four, and pause for a count of four. Then, repeat the cycle. The rhythmic nature of this pattern can help stabilize mood and increase focus, which makes it a valuable tool for moments of high stress or emotional overwhelm.

- **Cleansing Breaths:** Take a deep breath in, envisioning the inhalation of calmness and positivity, and then exhale fully, visualizing the release of tension and negativity. Cleansing breaths can be particularly effective in situations where quick emotional relief is needed.

Establish a Routine

Consistent meditation practice is necessary to reap the long-term benefits of mindfulness. Start by setting aside a specific time each day for meditation, even if it's just five to ten minutes. Consistency is more important than duration, and regular practice will help make meditation a natural part of your daily routine. Find a quiet space where you won't be disturbed, and make it your designated meditation spot. Over time, your brain will associate this space with relaxation and mindfulness, making slipping into a meditative state easier.

It's also helpful to add mindfulness to everyday activities. Practice mindful eating by paying full attention to your food's taste, texture, and aroma. Turn mundane tasks like washing dishes or sweeping the floor into opportunities for mindfulness by focusing entirely on the sensations involved.

These small, intentional acts of mindfulness add up over time and create a more grounded and present state of being.

As you get into mindfulness and meditation, approach these practices with patience and self-compassion. There will be days when distractions seem insurmountable or emotional discomfort arises. Accept these experiences without judgment and view them as part of the learning process. Remember, the goal of mindfulness is not to eliminate thoughts or emotions but to change your relationship with them.

Guided Meditation Resources

There is an abundance of guided meditation resources that make the practice of meditation less intimidating and more accessible. These resources cater specifically to those new to meditation by providing clear instructions and support, which allows you to focus on your experience without feeling lost or overwhelmed. With a variety of themes available, such as stress relief, anxiety reduction, or emotional healing, guided meditations can address specific emotional needs, help you connect with your feelings, and assist in finding solace. Adding audio-visual components enriches the meditation experience by creating a more engaging and immersive environment. It can help you feel more relaxed and present. This multi-sensory approach encourages you to embrace meditation as a beneficial daily practice. A quick search on your chosen app store or the internet will provide several options for guided meditations.

Set and Achieve Personal Goals

As you heal and empower yourself, setting personal goals that resonate with your inner needs and aspirations becomes important. When you define and reach these goals effectively, you develop a path of continuous growth and emotional balance.

Identify What Truly Matters

The first step in your goal-setting process is to understand what truly matters to you. Reflect on your values, passions, and the aspects of life that bring you joy and fulfillment. Ask yourself questions like:

- What makes me feel alive?

- What activities or achievements fill me with a sense of purpose?

Dig deep into your past experiences and identify moments when you felt most connected to your true self.

Journaling can be an invaluable tool in this exploration. Write about your dreams, fears, and desires without judgment to help you uncover patterns and insights that reveal your core values. If you struggle with this introspective process, consider seeking support from a mental health practitioner or coach who can guide you through exercises designed to improve self-awareness and clarity.

Establish SMART Goals

Once you have a clearer understanding of what matters most to you, it's time to translate these insights into actionable goals. The SMART methodology provides a structured approach to goal-setting, ensuring that your objectives are specific, measurable, achievable, relevant, and time-bound.

- **Specific:** Clearly articulate your objective. Rather than simply stating, "I want to heal my inner child," define what that means to you. For instance, "I intend to journal weekly to explore and nurture my past experiences."

- **Measurable:** Identify concrete metrics to assess your progress. This might include the amount of time dedicated to self-reflection each week, the number of journaling entries completed, or the frequency of practicing self-compassion exercises.

- **Achievable:** Formulate attainable goals that push you yet remain realistic. Aiming to completely resolve childhood issues in a month may be impractical if you're just beginning this journey. Instead, focus on identifying and addressing one specific memory at a time.

- **Relevant:** Ensure your objectives align with your deeper values and long-term aspirations. Reflect on why healing your inner child is essential and how it supports your overall emotional health.

- **Time-bound:** Establish a deadline for your healing process or parts of it. Setting a specific timeframe instills a sense of urgency and keeps you motivated. For example, "I will complete my first set of reflective journaling prompts within the next four weeks."

Include your inner child in the goal-setting process to increase your motivation by tapping into the inherent curiosity, creativity, and joy that characterize childhood. It helps you reconnect with your authentic desires and dreams, which are often overshadowed by adult responsibilities and societal expectations. If you allow your inner child to influence the goal-setting process, you can set goals that resonate with your true passions and interests, making the pursuit more exciting and fulfilling. This playful engagement creates a sense of adventure and wonder, which can reignite your motivation and enthusiasm, as you are more inclined to pursue goals that align with your genuine self rather than those dictated by external pressures.

Acknowledge Achievements

No matter how small, it's important to celebrate your accomplishments to maintain motivation and reinforce positive behaviors. Each achievement, big or small, marks progress on your healing journey and should be recognized and valued.

Create a system for acknowledging your milestones. This could be a gratitude journal where you record daily or weekly achievements or a visual tracker like a progress chart. Share your successes with friends or family members who support your journey. These celebrations boost your morale and create a positive feedback loop that encourages continued effort.

Find Accountability Partners

Accountability partners can help you stay committed to your goals. These partners can be friends, family members, or professionals like coaches or therapists who provide encouragement, feedback, and a sense of responsibility. Choose someone who understands your background and values your goals. Regular check-ins, whether weekly coffee meetings or virtual chats, can give you the necessary support and motivation to continue healing. Discuss your goals openly with your partner, sharing both your challenges and successes. They will support you and celebrate with you.

Healthy Habits for Maintaining Emotional Balance

Daily habits are important to achieving emotional balance and conscious living. These habits support our mental and emotional well-being, which helps heal the inner child. Your diet, exercise, sleep, and self-reflection are necessary for good emotional health.

Nutrition and Mood

Diet influences emotional health, as the foods we consume can affect our mood and overall mental well-being. Certain nutrients, such as omega-3 fatty acids, vitamins, and minerals, are needed for brain function and emotional regulation (Selhub, 2022). For instance, diets rich in whole grains, fruits, and vegetables provide the necessary vitamins and antioxidants that support brain health and reduce inflammation, which is linked to mood disorders. Conversely, a diet high in processed foods, sugars, and unhealthy fats can lead to unstable blood sugar levels and increased anxiety, thus adversely impacting emotional stability.

Nutritional choices have a huge effect on mood and energy levels, directly influencing how we feel throughout the day. Eating balanced meals that include a variety of nutrients can help keep steady energy levels and prevent mood swings. For example, complex carbohydrates found in whole grains help increase serotonin levels, a neurotransmitter associated with feelings of happiness and well-being. Similarly, proteins rich in tryptophan, such as turkey and nuts, also contribute to serotonin production (Watson, 2023). If you prioritize nutrient-dense foods, you can improve your mood, boost energy levels, and improve your emotional resilience.

Mindful eating also creates a stronger connection to bodily needs. You should be present during meals and pay attention to hunger cues so you can learn to honor your body's signals and adopt healthier eating habits. Mindful eating focuses on whole foods and hydration while advocating for moderation in consuming processed foods and alcohol. This awareness makes food more enjoyable and helps you develop a more compassionate relationship with your body. As a result, mindfulness eating practices can contribute to your overall emotional health and well-being, which enables you to make conscious choices that positively impact your mental state.

Physical Activity

Exercise is another vital part of emotional well-being. Regular physical activity releases endorphins, which are natural mood lifters. Exercise can help reduce stress, improve sleep, and increase overall happiness (Tartakovsky, 2022). Doing physical activity has been shown to improve cognitive functions and alleviate symptoms of anxiety and depression (West, 2022). Regular exercise creates a sense of accomplishment and increases self-esteem, so you feel more in control of your emotions and well-being. Make exercise a consistent part of your lifestyle to experience better mental clarity, more focus, and improved resilience against the challenges of everyday life.

One of the main reasons exercise is a natural mood enhancer is through the release of endorphins, often called the "feel-good" hormones. Physical activity signals your body to release these chemicals that act as natural painkillers and mood lifters (Tartakovsky, 2022). This phenomenon is commonly associated with the "runner's high," but it applies to various forms of exercise. Even moderate exercises such as walking or dancing can lead to increased happiness and a more positive outlook on life. Regularly experiencing these endorphin boosts can motivate you to create a sustainable fitness routine that benefits your mental health.

If you're new to exercising or have physical limitations, try low-impact activities such as yoga or stretching. These activities can help improve flexibility, reduce tension, and increase relaxation. Even short exercise sessions can make a huge difference in your mental health. Find enjoyable physical activities to stick to your fitness routine more easily, as enjoyment can drive commitment. When you do activities you love—whether it's cycling, swimming, or yoga—you're more likely to keep up with your regimen. Group activities can also add social support and connection, which further increases motivation. Exercising with friends or in community classes creates a sense of belonging and accountability, which makes workouts feel less like a chore and more like a rewarding social experience. The combination of enjoyment and social interaction keeps you active and contributes positively to your mental well-being.

Sleep Hygiene

Quality sleep is essential for emotional health because a lack of sleep can lead to increased feelings of stress, anxiety, and depression (Peri, 2021). To develop healthy sleep patterns, establish a consistent sleep schedule by going to bed and waking up at the same time every day. This helps regulate your body's internal clock, which makes it easier to fall asleep and wake up naturally.

A relaxing bedtime routine can tell your body it's time to wind down. This might include reading a book, taking a warm bath, or practicing deep-breathing exercises. Avoid screens—such as phones, tablets, and televisions—at least an hour before bed, as the blue light emitted can interfere with your ability to fall asleep.

You can also make your bedroom a sleep-friendly environment. Keep it cool, dark, and quiet, and invest in a comfortable mattress and pillows. Avoid caffeine and heavy meals close to bedtime, as they can disrupt your sleep. If you experience ongoing sleep issues, talk to a healthcare professional; they can better assist you.

Daily Check-Ins

We've already discussed how self-reflection can help you understand and manage your emotions, but it's worth touching on again. A daily ritual of self-reflection can help you become more aware of your emotional states and identify patterns or triggers.

Set aside a few minutes each day to reflect on your emotions. You might choose to do this in the morning, evening, or during a quiet moment in your day. Find a comfortable space where you won't be disturbed, and consider using a journal to record your thoughts and feelings.

In your self-reflection practice, ask yourself questions such as:

- What emotions am I experiencing right now?

- What events or interactions might have triggered these emotions?

- How did I respond to these emotions?

- What can I learn from this experience?

Be honest with yourself, and recognize both positive and negative emotions without judgment. Over time, this practice can help you gain insight into your emotional patterns and develop healthier ways of coping with difficult feelings.

Think about adding mindfulness techniques to your self-reflection ritual. Practices like meditation or deep-breathing exercises can help calm your mind and create a sense of inner peace. Mindfulness encourages you to stay present in the moment and reduces rumination about past events or worries about the future.

Coping Strategies for Stressful Moments

It is important to have a toolkit of practical and actionable techniques to manage stress and emotional triggers effectively. These strategies can help you create a more balanced and resilient approach to your everyday life.

Grounding Techniques

Learning to return focus to the present moment is an effective stress management technique. Grounding techniques anchor our thoughts and emotions to the here and now. They can be as easy as focusing on your breath or doing sensory activities like touching cold water or holding an object with a distinct texture. These practices help reduce the impact of overwhelming emotions by diverting your attention away from distressing thoughts and bringing your mind back to what is immediate and tangible.

Grounding exercises are practical tools for quickly diffusing feelings of panic or overwhelm, helping you regain a sense of control and stability in the face of anxiety. You can use grounding exercises to create a physical and mental anchor that can help calm racing thoughts and reduce the intensity of your emotional distress. The idea is to focus on your immediate surroundings.

A popular grounding technique is the "5-4-3-2-1" method, which uses mindfulness to engage the senses and increase your awareness of the present. In this exercise, you identify five things you can see, four things you can touch, three things you can hear, two things you can smell, and one thing you can taste. Using your senses intentionally distracts you from emotional turmoil and restores a sense of calmness.

Positive Distractions

Healthy distractions can also help during moments of distress. When you experience intense emotions, doing activities like reading a book, watching a favorite TV show, or practicing a hobby can provide much-needed relief. These activities are positive diversions and allow your mind to take a break from stressors. It's essential to choose enjoyable and fulfilling distractions rather than those that might lead to avoidance or procrastination.

Activities that involve music, art, or physical movement will help to shift your focus away from stressors. Listening to music can evoke positive emotions and create a soothing atmosphere, while creating art is an outlet for self-expression and emotional release. Physical activity, including structured workouts or taking a walk, promotes physical health and triggers the release of endorphins, which further reduces feelings of distress. Using creativity as a means of expression, such as journaling or painting, offers a therapeutic avenue to process emotions and find clarity, empowering you to work through your feelings constructively. Healthy distractions can nurture resilience and improve your ability to deal with stress, so incorporate them into your day where necessary.

Emotional Regulation Techniques

You may require specific tools and techniques to deal with intense emotions and become more resilient. For instance, recognizing and labeling emotions can help you understand your feelings without becoming overwhelmed by them. Cognitive reframing is another technique where you challenge negative thought patterns and replace them with more balanced perspectives. For example, instead of thinking, "I can't handle this," you could reframe it to, "This is tough, but I can find a way through it."

If you understand your emotions, you can identify specific triggers that lead to intense emotional responses. Once these triggers are recognized, you can create a proactive plan that makes you more prepared and allows you to anticipate and respond to challenges more effectively. This level of awareness empowers you to manage your emotions and gives you a sense of agency over your emotional experiences.

Practical strategies, like breathing techniques or visualization exercises, can effectively calm your mind and reduce overwhelming feelings. Simple breathing exercises, like deep diaphragmatic breathing, help lower heart rates and reduce stress levels by increasing relaxation. Visualization strategies, where you imagine serene and comforting environments, can further shift your focus away from distressing thoughts and provide a sense of tranquility. Self-soothing techniques—such as doing comforting activities, using positive affirmations, or listening to calming music—allow you to develop inner peace. These emotional regulation techniques can improve your ability to cope with life's challenges, leading to improved emotional well-being and a greater sense of balance in your life.

Seek Support

It's important to reach out for help during difficult times. Look for support from friends, family, or mental health professionals who can provide emotional relief and practical advice. Asking for help is a strength, not a weakness. Professional resources, such as counseling or therapy, offer safe spaces to explore emotions and develop customized strategies for managing stress. In addition to professional help, community resources and helplines can also be valuable. Every country has mental health organizations that can support and guide you during emotional difficulties. These services provide confidential assistance and can be a lifeline during challenging times.

Consistency in Practicing New Behaviors

Developing and maintaining new positive behaviors is crucial for emotional healing. Living with past trauma or emotional neglect often leads to patterns that no longer serve us well. It can be challenging to change these habits, but it is essential to develop a healthier and more balanced life.

Build New Routines

New practices can initially seem overwhelming, but breaking them down into manageable steps can make the process smoother. For example, start by identifying one positive behavior you want to adopt, such as practicing gratitude. Instead of aiming for a complete transformation overnight, begin with small actions like writing down three things you're thankful for each morning. This practice will become part of your routine over time, and its benefits will add up.

To make the process less daunting, consider adding techniques gradually. Start with something that feels most accessible to you. Perhaps focus on mindfulness practices if they resonate more with your current lifestyle. Techniques like mindful breathing can be easily incorporated into everyday activities. When feeling overwhelmed, taking a few deep breaths and centering yourself can help manage stress effectively. You could also decide to focus on physical or group activities if that appeals to you. Whatever you choose to do will have a positive impact on your emotional resilience.

Use Reminders

It's normal to struggle with sticking to new habits, so you may want to use reminders. Reminders can be tailored to your preferences to add an element of personalization to your healing process. For instance, creating a vision board can be a continual source of inspiration if you are visually oriented. On the other hand, if you respond better to auditory cues, recording affirmations and playing them during specific times of the day might be more effective. The idea is to choose methods that resonate with you personally to ensure consistency and engagement.

Visual aids, such as sticky notes on your bathroom mirror or refrigerator, can serve as prompt reminders of your intended positive actions. Similarly, setting alarms or notifications on your phone can reinforce your commitment. These reminders keep your goals at the forefront of your mind and provide a consistent nudge toward progress.

The Power of Reflection

Regular self-evaluation helps you identify your progress and areas that need more attention. A simple yet effective way to do this is by journaling. Regularly noting down your thoughts, experiences, and feelings creates a record of your journey. Over time, reviewing these entries enables you to see patterns and recognize how far you've come, which can boost your motivation and commitment to continue.

Any kind of self-assessment should be approached with kindness and patience. It's common to experience setbacks, but viewing these as learning opportunities rather than failures can make you more resilient. Establish a check-in schedule, perhaps weekly or monthly, to evaluate your progress. Take note of what worked well and where there were challenges. This reflective practice allows you to tweak your approach, making necessary adjustments and celebrating small improvements.

Celebrate Progress

Celebrate your achievements. Celebrations don't need to be grand; even small acknowledgments—such as treating yourself to a favorite activity or sharing your success with a friend—can be powerful motivators. Acknowledging milestones improves your self-belief and gives you a sense of accomplishment, which creates a positive reinforcement loop. This principle applies whether the milestones are related to your behavioral changes or broader life goals.

You can include your support network when celebrating achievements. Share your milestones with friends, family, or support groups to create a shared joy and reinforce your commitment through their encouragement. Collective celebrations increase the emotional impact of your progress and develop a supportive environment where people acknowledge every step forward, no matter how small.

You can also build a personalized rewards system. Tailor your rewards to match your interests and preferences. For instance, rewarding yourself with a new book or a relaxing bath after achieving a particular milestone can be highly motivating. This approach makes the process enjoyable and links positive experiences with your efforts, reinforcing the desire to continue.

Remember, developing new behaviors is not a linear process. It requires gradual change, marked by both triumphs and setbacks. Accept this reality with compassion toward yourself. Each step—even the tiny ones—contributes to the larger goal of emotional healing and well-being.

Heal Every Day

It's clear that everyday strategies and tools for healing can help you treat your inner child well. You can add techniques like mindfulness into your daily routine to improve your self-awareness and connect more deeply with your inner child. The various styles of meditation and breathing exercises are practical methods to calm the mind and body so that you get relief in moments of stress. The goal is progress, not perfection, but it allows you to gradually build a balanced and resilient emotional state for years to come.

9

STORIES OF TRANSFORMATION

Healing the inner child is a journey many undergo to transform their lives. By facing their past traumas and emotional wounds, they unlock pathways to self-love, personal growth, and resilience. In this chapter, we'll share the remarkable experiences of those who have taken this courageous step. We will see how they confronted childhood adversities, embraced their vulnerabilities, and made significant strides in healing.

Personal Narratives of Overcoming Trauma

Let's start by talking about the compelling paths some people have undertaken in search of healing their inner child. They confronted and overcame the shadows of childhood trauma, allowing for immense self-love and personal growth. Names have been changed to protect the identities of each person.

Resilience

The path to resilience often begins with overcoming neglect. William's story demonstrates how he sought help after years of emotional abandonment. It wasn't easy, and it required reaching out to supportive individuals such as therapists, mentors, and compassionate friends. This external support became a lifeline and allowed him to build resilience against the feelings of worthlessness instilled during his childhood. Through steadfast commitment to therapy and community support, William discovered the strength to rewrite his story, moving from a place of self-neglect to one of self-awareness and empowerment.

Healing

Embracing the wounded inner child means confronting painful memories head-on, which can be an intimidating task. Sophia knows this all too well. She grew up in a critical household where she didn't receive love and attention unless she performed well. This led to patterns of self-criticism and shame that had been imparted by her emotionally abusive parents. Sophia turned to journaling, meditation, and guided visualizations to extend compassion toward her younger self. These transformative moments were marked by the recognition of past hurts and an active choice to treat herself with kindness and empathy. Little by little, she peeled away layers of self-doubt and began to have more uplifting inner dialogue.

Joy

Bullying can create long-lasting wounds and embed a deep sense of inadequacy and fear. Mia's story illustrates how confronting these internalized fears through positive affirmations and cognitive behavioral techniques led to change. Mia learned to quiet the voices of past bullies by focusing on building a strong, compassionate, and validating inner voice. She participated in activities where she felt competent and valued, which bolstered her confidence. Mia celebrated each small victory in self-acceptance and reinforced her belief in her own abilities.

Forgiveness

Reconciliation with the past is another part of healing the inner child. Many find peace through forgiveness, which is both powerful and liberating. A particularly poignant story comes from Fletcher, who had harbored resentment and anger toward his neglectful caregivers. He attended forgiveness workshops and practiced mindfulness, gradually releasing these heavy emotions. This process didn't absolve his caregivers' actions but allowed him to reclaim his power by letting go of the grudges that had kept him tethered to the past. Forgiveness became a form of self-love for Fletcher, opening the door to emotional release and newfound freedom.

In each of these stories, the journey to healing and transformation is not linear. It has highs and lows—a testament to the complexity of dealing with childhood traumas. However, the common thread that runs through all these experiences is the undeniable impact of searching for help and extending compassion toward oneself. Supportive influences–whether they come from professional therapy, loved ones, or community groups–are vital components of these journeys.

Transformative moments are often characterized by a change in perception. For example, understanding that the critical inner voice–usually an echo of past abusers–is not an accurate reflection of one's worth can be revelatory. This newfound awareness can quicken the development of a kinder, more forgiving internal dialogue.

Another essential element in these stories is the act of celebrating small victories. Healing is about eradicating pain and acknowledging progress, however minor it may seem. Whether it's standing up to a critical family member, prioritizing self-care routines, or expressing emotions openly, each step forward is a triumph over past adversities.

These stories emphasize that while the journey to heal the inner child may begin with addressing neglect, abuse, or bullying, it ultimately leads to a fuller, more compassionate understanding of yourself. Reconciliation with the past does not mean forgetting or excusing it, but rather, finding a way to integrate those experiences into a broader story of growth and self-empowerment.

Lessons Learned From Different Experiences

Many of these stories share some common lessons. We may come from vastly different backgrounds or have experienced unique forms of trauma, but there are shared elements that shed light on human resilience and the non-linear paths to recovery.

Inherent Resilience

The inherent capacity for resilience found within each of us is a common theme. Despite our adversities, we often exhibit a remarkable ability to adapt, recover, and grow. Building resilience is filled with setbacks and progress. The healing process isn't straightforward; it is more of a winding road where moments of breakthrough are frequently followed by periods of struggle. This ebb and flow is natural and shows that healing is a dynamic and continuous process, not a destination.

Diversity of Healing

There is no single "correct" way to heal. Each person's path to self-love is valid and shaped by their personal experiences and the unique impact of their trauma. For some of us, healing may involve therapy and medication, while others might find solace in creative outlets or community support. These varying approaches show that healing is deeply personal. What works for one individual may not work for another, but every path is legitimate and deserves recognition. This diversity also highlights the importance of honoring your pace and methods of recovery, as everyone's experience with trauma and healing is unique yet valid.

Vulnerability Matters

The experiences shared in the first section emphasize the importance of vulnerability and creating safe spaces for the inner child. Allowing yourself to be vulnerable can be incredibly scary, especially if you have been hurt in the past. However, it is in these moments of openness that true healing begins. If you acknowledge and tend to the needs of your inner child, you can create a loving environment within yourself and enable growth and self-compassion. This internal safety allows for the exploration of deep-seated fears and wounds, which can lead to a personal transformation.

Empowerment

Sharing stories of transformation and healing is an essential tool for our community. Individuals who share their experiences empower themselves and encourage others to continue their healing journeys. We can vocalize struggles and triumphs so others realize they are not alone in their experiences. This collective sharing creates a sense of community and belonging, which is essential for emotional recovery.

Are you ready to share your story? Start by reflecting on your journey and identifying key moments of change or realization. Write these down and focus on how you felt and responded to these events. When you're ready, share your story with a trusted friend, family member, therapist, or support group. Remember to be gentle with yourself throughout this process, as revisiting past traumas can be challenging. Your story has the potential to inspire and heal both you and those who hear it. Empowerment through storytelling creates a ripple effect, facilitates healing on a larger scale, and contributes to a culture of openness and support.

Impact of Healing on Personal Growth

Healing can help you grow in ways you never imagined possible. You will discover new things about yourself, your abilities, and your remarkable resiliency.

Rediscovering Your Identity

Changing how we see ourselves after healing can be an important journey that helps people grow beyond their past struggles. Healing the inner child means recognizing and dealing with past hurts, which often changes how we view ourselves. For example, someone who felt unwanted or unworthy as a child may start to believe they deserve love and can achieve great things. This change leads to a new sense of identity, where a person's self-worth is shaped by their current strengths and goals rather than their past pain.

After facing your painful past, you can find your identity. Healing requires getting over trauma or emotional pain before experiencing personal growth. As you explore your past experiences, you may discover parts of yourself that you had hidden or ignored. This process can lead to important insights about your values, interests, and goals, which allow you to redefine who you are. Reflect on your thoughts and feelings, and you will gain a renewed sense of purpose and direction, which will give you a more profound and better understanding of yourself.

Self-discovery after healing can be very empowering. It shows how you can change and grow by embracing your stories. By facing your past, you can better understand what matters to you, which helps you know who you are. This change allows you to move past the labels and expectations given to you by society or yourself and opens up new possibilities. As you redefine who you are, you learn to be kind to yourself and take control of your lives, thriving in ways you never thought possible. The healing process turns pain into strength, leading to a new identity that shows resilience, authenticity, and a strong belief in your potential.

Better Relationships

Working on your inner child can lead to better relationships. Understanding and working through your past issues teaches you to set better boundaries and communicate well. For example, someone who used to accept bad behavior from others because they didn't value themselves might now feel strong enough to express their needs. This improves current relationships and helps you form healthier ones in the future. Because you have worked on your inner child, you can spot harmful patterns and make choices that encourage respect and support.

Working on your inner child teaches you more about yourself, including your needs, wants, and emotional triggers. This new understanding helps you interact with others in a kinder way, which leads to healthier relationships based on trust and understanding. As you heal, you can connect with others honestly and form bonds built on love and respect.

The inner child healing process teaches us how crucial it is to set boundaries and build respect in relationships. When you recognize your worth and learn to care for yourself, you become better at sharing your needs and expectations. This change improves your interactions with others and encourages those around you to respect these boundaries. Harmful relationships can become supportive ones, indicating the growth that comes from inner child work. Instead of getting caught up in manipulation or fights, your relationships can thrive through clear communication, understanding, and commitment. It creates a safe environment where you feel valued and supported, which leads to deeper, more meaningful connections that improve your life.

Emotional Autonomy

Personal stories about gaining emotional independence after healing show significant changes in people's lives as they learn to manage their feelings. It helps you learn to manage your feelings and accept them without needing the approval of others. Being able to control your emotions is vital for personal growth because it helps you face life's challenges calmly instead of acting impulsively.

This process often starts with understanding how to control your emotions, which helps you deal with your feelings without being overwhelmed. As you heal, you may identify unhealthy patterns of being overly reliant on others and understand the need to take care of your emotional health. With a renewed focus on managing emotions, you can change how you interact with yourself and others.

You will change when you learn to value your feelings and rely less on what others think. Instead of looking for approval from others, you will find strength in recognizing and accepting your emotions. This change builds your confidence as you better understand and learn to express your emotional needs. As you develop your independence, you create healthier relationships and boost your self-worth. The path to emotional independence involves personal growth and learning about yourself, which helps you accept who you are so you can face the world with new strength and clarity.

Pursuit of Passions

One of the most rewarding outcomes of healing your inner child is the ability to follow your passions. Once you reconnect with your inner child, you may rediscover hobbies and interests you had forgotten. This connection can spark more creativity and happiness. Doing activities that bring you joy, like painting, writing, or dancing, becomes a way to express your newfound freedom and self-awareness. Exploring and pursuing these interests usually leads to a more vibrant life filled with real moments of happiness.

Healing helps you let go of fears and self-doubt that limit your ability to fully enjoy these passions, leading you to choose paths that are both fulfilling and true to who you are. The link between personal growth and the freedom to follow your passions becomes clear as you shed limiting beliefs and societal expectations that have shaped your identity. A newfound sense of freedom creates an environment where you can explore and try new things.

Key Turning Points in The Healing Journey

Some key moments in the process of healing your inner child can lead to important changes and growth. These moments help you see things differently and allow you to think about your life and notice the turning points that guide you toward healing.

Moments of Awakening

Many people have moments of realization during times of deep thinking or after major life events, and you may, too. For example, someone might suddenly understand how harmful habits like drinking too much alcohol can be. After many mornings filled with regret and feeling embarrassed in social situations, they might finally choose to change their behavior and look for a happier and more meaningful life because they realize drinking alcohol is a coping mechanism. These moments are necessary and can lead to greater self-discovery and understanding.

Support Networks

Support networks are crucial for change. Healing is rarely done alone. Community, like family, friends, or support groups, all play an important role. These groups provide safe spaces to share experiences, connect emotionally, and build strength together. They reflect your individual progress and offer comfort during tough times. Think of someone who has struggled alone for years and finally talks to a trusted group about their struggles; they may find many others have experienced the same thing. Sharing can reduce feelings of loneliness and strengthen their commitment to healing. Support networks help everyone grow together; when one person heals, they often inspire others in the group, creating a strong sense of community and support.

More Emotional Vulnerability

Another part of healing is accepting emotional vulnerability. Being vulnerable takes courage but is necessary for real healing. It means letting yourself feel and show deep emotions without worrying about being judged. For example, someone might go to therapy and share painful childhood memories for the first time. Through this, they realize that vulnerability is not a weakness but a strength that helps them better understand their emotions. This honesty helps build trust with themselves and others, which is essential for personal growth. Vulnerability, then, opens the door to new strength and resilience.

Committing to Change

Commitments to change are the steps people take to make important changes in their lives after realizing something significant. These commitments are necessary because they turn ideas and thoughts into actual plans and help you keep going on your journey to change. For example, someone might start going to yoga or practicing mindfulness. This helps them exercise and improves their mental focus and emotional balance.

Daily commitments can also help you heal. Each small step helps with the larger goal of knowing and loving yourself, which helps you form new habits that improve your well-being over time. Committing to change often means setting clear and realistic goals. These goals can include finding better ways to handle stress, building supportive relationships, or spending time every day on activities that boost your mental and emotional health. Sticking to these commitments helps create a clear path to healing and makes your personal growth feel real and achievable.

Finding Inspiration

Starting a healing journey can be challenging, but it can also change your life. The stories shared at the beginning of the chapter demonstrate that. They are packed with lessons and inspiration that can motivate your healing process.

Empowerment and Hope

Empowerment and hope are essential parts of any story about change. Small actions can lead to big changes, as shown by many people who have faced tough times. Something small, like taking just five minutes a day to meditate, can grow into a daily routine of self-care that changes your life. Each little you take will strengthen you and give you the ability to cope.

Similarly, changing your mindset can lead to fundamental changes. You might be stuck in self-doubt and fear because of past trauma, but you can decide to challenge your negative thoughts with positive affirmations. At first, you may be skeptical, but keep trying anyway. Over time, this practice can change how you talk to yourself, raising your confidence and giving you hope for the future. These simple changes show that empowerment can grow slowly and provide hope for those who feel lost in their healing process.

Self-Compassion

Self-compassion is imperative for taking care of your inner child. It means treating yourself with the same kindness you would show to a good friend. To care for your inner child, start by being kind to yourself. This could mean speaking softly to yourself, allowing yourself to rest without feeling guilty, or doing things just for fun. Practices like mindfulness, where you pay attention to your thoughts and feelings without being too hard on yourself or writing in a journal, can help you understand and accept yourself better. By seeing your struggles as common to everyone, you learn to forgive yourself for your flaws and mistakes. Simple self-care activities like walking in nature, enjoying a relaxing bath, or reading a favorite book can also help strengthen self-compassion.

Take Action

You need to do something to heal your inner child; it won't happen on its own. Taking action is important for implementing these ideas in everyday life. Tools like meditation apps, self-help books, or support groups can offer help. Activities like deep breathing, keeping a gratitude journal, or setting limits can also fit into your daily activities. Adding these easy but valuable habits can lead to lasting improvement.

Connect Through Community

Community and connection are important for healing and emphasize the value of sharing stories and seeking support. Connecting with others who have similar experiences can help you feel accepted and understood. Support groups, whether in person or online, provide safe spaces for you to tell your stories and gain encouragement.

After feeling alone because of your trauma for years, you may find comfort and strength by meeting others who understand your suffering. A supportive atmosphere allows you to talk about your feelings freely and helps you heal more quickly. You can speak openly about their experiences, build connections, and support each other in healing. Healing is not done alone; it grows with the understanding and compassion of others.

Write Your Story

This chapter shares the journeys of people who are healing from their childhood experiences and learning to love themselves. You are part of these stories. Each story shows how important it is to get help and to be kind to yourself. Through therapy, community support, and practices like writing in a journal and meditation, you can change your stories, moving from neglect and harsh self-judgment to feeling empowered and caring for yourself. Healing has ups and downs, with small wins and big changes. But even though the journey can be tough, it leads to a better understanding and more compassion for yourself.

10

Achieve Lasting
Emotional Freedom

To achieve lasting emotional freedom, you need to combine mindfulness with daily habits that help you heal in all areas of your life. Small, purposeful changes—such as focusing more on your daily activities or regularly checking in with your feelings—can lead to ongoing well-being. Staying present and understanding your emotions builds a stronger and more balanced inner life.

Integrating Lessons Into Daily Life

How do you add these positive habits to your day-to-day activities? We've already discussed several strategies in previous chapters, but let's take some time now to consider some more practical ways to do inner child work daily.

Focus on Mindfulness Integration

Mindfulness can be added to everyday tasks to transform mundane routines into emotional healing and growth opportunities. For example, think about your morning routine. Instead of rushing through brushing your teeth or making coffee, take a few moments to focus on the sensations involved. Notice the texture of the toothbrush against your teeth, the taste of toothpaste, and the warmth of the water as it flows over your hands. This simple act of paying attention can ground you in the present moment, reduce stress, and give you a sense of calm. Regular mindfulness can reduce anxiety, improve mood, and increase emotional resilience.

Routine Check-Ins

Routine check-ins are another valuable tool for maintaining emotional freedom. Regularly assess your emotional state to improve your self-awareness and address issues before they escalate. Set aside a few minutes each day for an emotional check-in. Ask yourself questions like, "How am I feeling right now?" or "What emotions have I experienced today?" These reflections can help you identify patterns in your emotional responses and understand what triggers positive and negative feelings. Remember to practice self-compassion as you do these check-ins.

Journaling can be an effective method for these check-ins. Write down your thoughts and emotions to create a tangible record of your emotional journey. It can help you process experiences and provide insights into your behavior. For those new to journaling, start with simple prompts such as

"What made me smile today?" or "What challenged me today?" As you become more comfortable, dig deeper into your emotions and explore both joys and frustrations.

Use Affirmations

Positive affirmations can challenge negative thoughts and give you a positive mindset, so they are valuable tools to combat negative self-talk and boost self-esteem. Create a list of affirmations that resonate with you, such as "I am worthy of love and happiness," "I am strong and capable," or "I am enough just as I am."

Start your day by repeating affirmations to yourself in the mirror or write them down and place them where you'll see them frequently, like on your computer screen or refrigerator. These positive messages can reshape your thought patterns and help you develop a more compassionate and supportive inner dialogue. You can also repeat them during your lunch break, before you go to bed, or any time you feel you need to lift your spirits.

Look for Joy

Find joyful moments throughout your day to help you achieve emotional balance. Do activities that bring you joy and make you feel alive and fulfilled. It could be anything from painting, gardening, dancing, or spending time in nature.

Make a conscious effort to incorporate these activities into your daily or weekly schedule. Even small doses of joy can greatly affect your emotional health. For instance, if you enjoy reading, set aside 15 minutes daily to immerse yourself in a good book. If you love being outdoors, plan regular walks in the park or hikes in nature. These moments of joy become emotional anchors that provide stability and contentment amidst life's challenges.

It's also beneficial to cultivate gratitude as part of this practice. Gratitude shifts your focus from what's wrong in your life to what's going well, giving you a positive outlook. Take time each day to reflect on things you're thankful for—big or small. It could be a supportive friend, a beautiful sunset, or a personal achievement. Regularly acknowledging these positives creates a reservoir of happiness and resilience to draw upon during tough times.

Continued Self-Growth and Reflection

Lifelong self-discovery and growth are important to achieving lasting emotional freedom. The process does not end with the initial healing; instead, it becomes an ongoing process of setting new goals, seeking feedback, and creating a growth mindset.

Set New Goals

Personal and emotional goals nurture proactive growth and propel us forward on our healing journey. After the initial wave of healing, it's essential to identify new aspirations that align with your evolving values and desires. These goals help maintain a sense of direction and purpose, which prevents complacency. For instance, you might set a goal to improve your communication skills to improve relationships or perhaps aim to start a new hobby that brings joy and fulfillment. These goals should align with the SMART framework we discussed in Chapter 8. Break down your goals into manageable steps and celebrate small victories along the way to reinforce your progress and commitment to continual self-improvement.

Seek Feedback

Feedback from friends, family, or professionals can give you invaluable perspectives that can help you identify blind spots that you would otherwise overlook. Constructive feedback helps to improve your self-awareness and encourages you to refine your behaviors and approaches. It's beneficial to create a supportive network of individuals whose opinions you value and trust. Regularly ask for their input on how you handle situations, manage emotions, or approach challenges. It will solidify your relationships and create a culture of open communication and mutual growth. Use feedback as a tool for learning rather than criticism, and recognize its potential to foster deep introspection and real change.

Participate in Workshops

Workshops or group therapy sessions provide a platform for fresh insights and connecting with others on similar journeys. These environments are opportunities to explore new strategies for coping, healing, and growing emotionally. Workshops designed around personal development, emotional regulation, or mindfulness can introduce innovative techniques to add to your daily life.

For example, a workshop on resilience might teach you valuable skills for bouncing back from adversity, while a mindfulness seminar might give you practice for staying present and calm. The collective experience shared within these groups can be immensely validating and help you realize that you are not alone in your struggles and triumphs. The structure of these sessions often includes interactive elements like role-playing or guided discussions, which can deepen your understanding and application of the concepts discussed. Participation accelerates your own growth and contributes positively to the group, which creates a sense of community and shared progress.

Adopt a Growth Mindset

A growth mindset—believing that abilities and intelligence can be developed through dedication and hard work—is necessary for continuous improvement and resilience. This mindset shifts the focus from looking for validation to using learning and viewing challenges as opportunities to grow rather than obstacles to avoid.

A growth mindset invites us to be curious about our limitations and failures, seeing them as stepping stones rather than setbacks. Instead of feeling defeated by a mistake, someone with a growth mindset would analyze the error, take lessons from it, and apply those lessons moving forward. It's an approach that builds resilience and enables us to persevere in the face of difficulties.

To nurture a growth mindset, regularly remind yourself that effort leads to success. Celebrate your progress and be patient with your development. Surround yourself with individuals who encourage this perspective and challenge you to strive for continual improvement. This mindset also helps with flexibility and allows you to adapt to changing circumstances without losing sight of your goals. You will be better equipped to deal with life's unpredictability and turn potential roadblocks into opportunities for advancement.

Celebrate Progress and Milestones

Recognizing and celebrating emotional progress is an essential part of healing your inner child. It validates your personal growth and motivates you to put in a continuous effort.

Establish Milestones

Milestones can help you achieve sustained progress. Milestones are specific, measurable goals that represent your main points of progress. These can be as basic as successfully using a new coping skill for a week or more complex, like maintaining consistent self-care routines over several months. Break down your larger goals into smaller, more achievable tasks to help establish milestones. For example, if improving self-confidence is the goal, initial milestones could include practicing positive self-talk daily or doing social activities once a week. Reaching these smaller targets can give you a sense of accomplishment that fuels your motivation to continue chasing your goals.

Measurable milestones give you a structured approach to healing. Begin by identifying specific areas needing improvement, such as reducing negative thought patterns or building healthier relationships. Then, break these broader goals into smaller, easily manageable tasks. For instance, if the overarching goal is to improve your relationship skills, a milestone could be having meaningful conversations with loved ones twice a week. These milestones should be clear and attainable, providing a road map that guides you step-by-step. As you reach each small milestone, you take another step closer to success. Celebrate these milestones and the positive behaviors required to meet them, which will make it more likely to stay committed to your emotional health.

Journal About Achievements

A journal can be an effective way to stay motivated because it helps to write down your thoughts, feelings, and progress on your emotional journey. This habit gives a clear record of your growth and makes it easier to see how much you have changed. For instance, writing about how you handled a tough situation today compared to six months ago can show big changes in your emotional strength. Also, reading past journal entries during hard times can provide comfort and motivation.

Regular journaling helps with self-reflection, which is important for better understanding your emotions. As you consistently write about your achievements, you start to see patterns in your behavior and feelings. This awareness improves your ability to handle challenges; over time, your journal becomes a valuable record of personal growth.

Share Successes

Sharing successes with others amplifies your sense of achievement, strengthens your connections, and provides validation. When you share your progress, whether with friends, family, or support groups, you receive positive reinforcement and encouragement, which creates a sense of community and belonging. For instance, discussing your personal victories in a therapy group can inspire others while also reaffirming your progress. The act of sharing can inspire others who are on similar journeys. Hearing about someone else's progress can provide hope and motivation, just like your story can inspire someone else. It reinforces the idea that emotional freedom is possible through perseverance and effort.

Create Rituals

Creating rituals for celebrating milestones is an intimate and personalized way to honor your progress. Rituals provide a structured yet flexible way to acknowledge your achievements. Personal rituals can vary widely depending on your preferences and values. They can be simple or elaborate, solitary or shared, but their central purpose is to create a moment of intentional reflection and celebration. For example, you could light a candle, meditate, or organize a small gathering with friends.

Adding rituals into your daily life ensures that your emotional progress is continuously acknowledged and celebrated. You are validating your efforts and building a stronger foundation for ongoing healing and development. Rituals are a physical manifestation of your internal journey and mark the transition from one stage of healing to the next. For instance, you may have reached a milestone in managing your anxiety and choose to celebrate by planting a tree to symbolize your growth and stability.

Stay Committed to the Healing Journey

Healing your inner child requires a sustained commitment to the process. This commitment includes regular check-ins, building a support network, scheduling time for self-care, and accepting the journey of recovery, including its inevitable setbacks.

Regular Check-Ins

Regular check-ins with yourself can help you assess your emotional health. Just as you would with physical health, periodically evaluate your mental state to become aware of any changes or declines in your well-being. You can ask yourself how you feel physically and emotionally at different points during the day or take a more structured approach once a day. Keep a journal to document these feelings and to get insights into your emotional patterns and triggers. You may notice recurring themes or stressors that affect your emotional state, which allows you to address them proactively. Mindfulness practices can improve these check-ins by making you more attuned to the present moment and your internal experiences.

Rely on Your Support Network

Your support network can help you maintain long-term emotional freedom. Surround yourself with supportive individuals who understand and respect your healing process so that you achieve a sense of security and encouragement. Friends, family members, support groups, or even online communities can offer different perspectives and practical advice during tough times. Choosing people who focus on positivity and growth rather than those who are negative or discourage you is important.

Social interactions can distract you from negative thoughts and allow you to focus on others. Support systems work both ways, meaning you may sometimes help others, which can also be uplifting. When friends check in on you, like inviting you for a walk, or family members suggest a healthy meal, it often helps you feel better. Similarly, you can also strengthen the relationship by asking others to join you in your daily or weekly activities.

Prioritize Self-Care

Self-care should be viewed as a non-negotiable part of your routine. It includes a range of activities from basic needs like eating nutritious meals and getting adequate sleep, to more personal practices such as doing hobbies, taking long baths, reading, or spending time in nature. These activities nurture your body and mind, improving mood regulation and increasing overall happiness (Wooll, 2022). Self-care builds emotional resilience and makes it easier to face life's challenges. Regular self-care creates self-awareness, enabling you to better understand and manage your emotions. When self-care becomes a habit, it's easier to maintain emotional stability and fight off burnout or emotional exhaustion.

Embrace the Journey

Embrace the journey of healing with all its ups and downs. Setbacks are a natural part of any recovery process and should be seen as opportunities for growth rather than failures. Healing is not linear, so you need to have patience and compassion for yourself. Each setback can teach you something valuable about your triggers, coping mechanisms, and resilience.

Reflect frequently on episodes of struggle to reveal new strengths and insights. For instance, you might discover that a particular strategy you used was ineffective, prompting you to try a different approach next time. This also means celebrating small victories along the way to acknowledge your progress, reinforce positive behaviors, and boost motivation.

Create an environment where you feel safe to explore and express your emotions without judgment to properly experience growth and healing. This might involve setting boundaries with people who don't understand your journey or limiting exposure to stressful situations when possible. Additionally, professional help can play a huge part in your healing process. Consult therapists, counselors, or other mental health professionals to give you additional tools and perspectives for deeper healing. They can guide you through complex emotions, offer evidence-based techniques, and support you in developing a personalized plan for emotional wellness.

Future-Focused Mindset and Opportunities

It's essential to look forward with hope and openness to new experiences. Doing so can create opportunities for growth and healing, which makes the future bright.

Visualize Your Goals

A good way to build a positive mindset is by imagining your future goals. Visualization can improve your motivation and focus and help you move toward what you want to achieve. Create a mental picture of your goals to inspire you and guide your actions. This practice strengthens the belief that your goals are achievable and shows you the steps needed to get there.

Visualization can seem like daydreaming, but it requires active focus. You can use visualization to imagine a future where you have overcome your struggles and healed from trauma. Imagining success helps build confidence and aligns your thoughts and actions with goals. For visualization, consider a guided imagery exercise where you close your eyes and picture your ideal future in vivid detail. Immerse themselves in the sensory experience: What do you see, hear, feel, and even smell? A detailed visualization helps solidify the mental blueprint of your goals, which makes them more tangible and attainable.

Welcome Change

Change is inevitable, and your ability to adapt and find opportunities within change can affect your personal growth and well-being. Resistance to change often comes from fear and uncertainty, including remnants of past trauma or negative experiences. However, being ready for change allows you to view it as a source of opportunity rather than a threat. This change in perspective can be created through small, manageable steps. For instance, taking up a new hobby or pursuing an interest that has always intrigued you is a great way to embrace change. By doing so, you begin to build resilience and adaptability, which are essential qualities to deal with life's unpredictable nature. Start small, then keep going. Even little changes add up and make it easier to welcome unexpected changes.

Discover Passions

Find hobbies that your inner child likes to feel better emotionally. Try new activities to reconnect with your younger self since it's a part of you that is often forgotten because of past difficulties. Do things that bring you happiness and curiosity to bring back a sense of joy and excitement about life. These activities let you explore different sides of themselves that may have been held back. Rediscovering hobbies brings happiness and helps with healing by creating a safe space for self-exploration and expression.

To find your passion, try different activities without feeling pressured to commit. Be open-minded and enjoy the experience, which may lead to unexpected discoveries about what you truly love. You can keep a journal to record your feelings and experiences, noting which activities you enjoy the most.

Set Intentions

Intentions are another way to guide your decision-making positively. Unlike vague resolutions, setting intentions involves specific, actionable statements that outline how you intend to approach life and its challenges. Intentions provide direction and purpose, ensuring that your daily actions align with your long-term goals. For example, an intention to practice gratitude daily can lead to a more positive outlook on life and increase emotional resilience. When you set clear intentions, you create a roadmap for your behavior and choices, making staying focused and aligned with your goals easier. Intention-setting can be particularly beneficial as you heal from trauma, as it empowers you to take control of your journey and make conscious decisions that support your well-being.

A helpful exercise is to start each day with a morning intention-setting ritual. Write down an intention for the day ahead, focusing on aspects like kindness, patience, or mindfulness. Review these intentions at the end of the day to see how well you were able to stay aligned with your goals and identify areas for improvement.

Keep Going

In this chapter, we discussed the importance of using healing practices daily to maintain lasting emotional freedom. Many small practices help us stay grounded in the present and build resilience and self-awareness, which enables us to deal with life's challenges more easily. As you continue your healing journey, remember that consistency and commitment are crucial. Each small step you take contributes to your growth and emotional health. Keep using these tools; over time, you'll find yourself stronger, more self-compassionate, and capable of handling whatever comes your way.

CONCLUSION

Take a moment to reflect on the path you've taken to learn more about your inner child. You have navigated the difficult terrain of healing from childhood trauma and emotional neglect, reconnected with your inner child, and nurtured the parts of yourself that have longed for attention and care. Acknowledging your inner child is a symbolic gesture and an ongoing practice of self-awareness and self-compassion. Understanding the wounds from your past is a critical part of this process, but it is equally important to recognize the strength and resilience you carry within. You've taken immense steps towards reclaiming your story and shaping it into one of growth and recovery by facing these old pains head-on.

Think back to the brave decision you made to confront your past. It takes courage to dig into memories that may have been buried. You may have found new methods to explore, understand, and deal with your past. From journaling about your experiences to practicing daily affirmations and engaging in therapeutic exercises, each effort marks a milestone in your transformation. Celebrating these achievements is important, no matter how small they may seem. Every bit of progress is a testament to your determination and willingness to heal.

Self-compassion has been a recurring theme throughout this process and serves as the foundation for all healing work. Learning to love and forgive yourself is an ongoing challenge, particularly when confronting painful memories. Yet, through self-compassion, you begin to break down the negative beliefs instilled during childhood and replace them with a kinder, more supportive narrative.

It's important to remember that healing is not linear, and it does not have a definitive endpoint. There will be days filled with joy and discovery, and there will be moments of doubt and discomfort. Accepting this reality allows you to stay adaptable and committed to the process. The tools you've acquired throughout this book are meant to support you during both the highs and the lows, offering stability and comfort as you heal. These practical tools and exercises are integral tools you can incorporate into your daily life. They help build lasting emotional resilience and provide a framework for continuous personal growth.

As you look ahead, I invite you to envision your future self: a version of you, unburdened by past traumas and thriving with emotional clarity and self-love. Picture the dreams and goals that now seem achievable because you have begun to break free from the chains of old wounds. What would your life look like if you fully embraced your potential? What opportunities could you seize, and what relationships might flourish? This vision is a tangible possibility waiting to unfold with each step you take forward. Set new goals, maintain a growth mindset, and keep this vision alive to propel you toward a more fulfilled existence. Your commitment to this process is the key to turning these dreams into reality.

As we wrap up this book, let me leave you with an affirmation that encapsulates the core message we've uncovered throughout our time together: "I am worthy of love. I am capable of change. My past does not define my future." Hold these words close to your heart as a reminder of your inherent worth and the progress you've made. Your story is powerful, and sharing it can inspire others who are walking similar paths. That is also a reminder that you are not alone in this journey. There is a community of individuals who understand and share your struggles; they are ready to offer support and empathy. Reach out, share your experiences, and allow others to uplift you as you move forward. Together, we can become beacons of resilience and hope for other people who are busy with the process of healing their inner child.

May you continue to grow, thrive, and find deep, abiding peace within yourself. Remember, you have within you the strength to heal and the capacity for boundless love and joy. Keep moving forward, embrace each moment, and hold onto the knowledge that you deserve all the good that life has to offer.

If you found this book helpful, please leave a review on your preferred book platform so others can commence their healing journey.

GLOSSARY

- **Acceptance:** Embracing reality and acknowledging feelings or situations without resistance or judgment.
- **Active listening:** Participating fully in a conversation by paying attention, understanding, responding, and remembering what the speaker is saying.
- **Affirmations:** Positive statements that are repeated to challenge negative beliefs and encourage self-empowerment.
- **Anxiety:** A feeling of worry, nervousness, or unease about something with an uncertain outcome.
- **Art therapy:** A therapeutic practice that uses creative expression through art to improve mental health and emotional well-being.
- **Attachment patterns:** Recurring behaviors in relationships that stem from childhood experiences that impact adult connections.
- **Attachment styles:** The characteristic ways individuals relate to others in relationships, largely influenced by childhood experiences.
- **Authentic interactions:** Genuine and honest exchanges between individuals that create trust and connection.

- **Authenticity in relationships:** Being true to oneself in interactions with others through transparency and honesty.
- **Adult behavior:** Actions and reactions that reflect maturity and responsibility.
- **Adverse Childhood Experiences (ACEs):** Traumatic events occurring before age 18 that can impact an individual's emotional and physical health.
- **Body awareness:** The conscious understanding and recognition of bodily sensations, movements, and emotions.
- **Body scan meditation:** A mindfulness practice that involves mentally scanning the body for areas of tension to increase relaxation.
- **Boundaries:** Limits set to protect oneself physically, emotionally, and mentally in relationships.
- **Boundary setting:** The process of defining personal limits and communicating them to others.
- **Cognitive behavioral therapy (CBT):** A therapeutic approach that focuses on changing negative thought patterns to improve emotions and behaviors.
- **Cognitive distortions:** Incorrect thought patterns that can lead to misinterpretations of situations and contribute to negative emotions.
- **Cognitive reframing:** The practice of changing the way one perceives a thought or situation to alter emotional responses.
- **Compassion:** Empathetic concern for the suffering of others, coupled with a desire to help alleviate it.

- **Community:** A group of individuals connected by shared interests, values, or goals that offers support and belonging.
- **Constructive feedback:** Positive, helpful criticism improves one's work or behavior.
- **Curiosity:** A desire to learn and understand more about people, situations, or topics.
- **Creative therapies:** Therapeutic approaches that utilize artistic expression, such as art, music, or drama, for healing.
- **Daily routines:** Structured activities performed regularly that contribute to overall well-being.
- **Daily self-care rituals:** Consistent practices incorporated into daily life to maintain physical, emotional, and mental health.
- **Deep breathing exercises:** Breathing techniques used to promote relaxation and reduce stress.
- **Depression:** A persistent feeling of sadness and loss of interest that can affect daily functioning.
- **Emotional abandonment:** The feeling of being unrecognized and unsupported by those who are supposed to provide emotional care.
- **Emotional abuse:** A form of abuse involving manipulation or emotional harm, typically through verbal attacks or victimization.
- **Emotional autonomy:** The ability to regulate one's own emotions and maintain independence in emotional experiences.
- **Emotional balance:** A state of emotional stability where feelings are managed effectively and healthily.

- **Emotional detachment:** A coping mechanism where an individual distances themselves from emotional experiences to avoid pain.
- **Emotional dysregulation:** Inability to manage emotions effectively which leads to intense emotional reactions.
- **Emotional freedom:** The state of being unshackled from past emotional traumas and able to feel and express emotions freely.
- **Emotional healing:** The process of recovering from emotional wounds and trauma to achieve a better mental state.
- **Emotional health:** The state of one's emotional well-being, including the ability to cope with stress and relate to others.
- **Emotional literacy:** The ability to recognize, understand, and articulate one's own emotions and the emotions of others.
- **Emotional neglect:** The failure to provide emotional support or attention, leading to feelings of unworthiness or abandonment.
- **Emotional pain points:** Specific areas of emotional distress that can trigger negative feelings or behaviors.
- **Emotional protection:** Strategies used to safeguard oneself from emotional harm or distress.
- **Emotional recovery:** The process of healing from emotional trauma and restoring emotional well-being.
- **Emotional regulation:** The ability to manage and respond to emotional experiences in a healthy way.
- **Emotional responses:** Reactions to emotional stimuli, which can vary in intensity and appropriateness.

- **Emotional resilience:** The capacity to recover quickly from difficulties and adapt to change.
- **Emotional safety:** A secure environment where individuals can express their feelings without fear of judgment or backlash.
- **Emotional scars:** Lasting effects of significant emotional pain or trauma, often influencing future behavior.
- **Emotional triggers:** Stimuli that provoke intense emotional reactions based on past experiences.
- **Emotional validation:** Acknowledgment and acceptance of another person's feelings as real and important.
- **Emotional wounds:** Psychological injuries that can result from past trauma, leading to ongoing emotional pain.
- **Empathy:** The ability to understand and share the feelings of another which facilitates connection and support.
- **Empowerment:** The process of gaining confidence and strength to make choices and take control of one's life.
- **Family systems:** The interconnected relationships and dynamics within a family unit that influence individual development.
- **Goals setting:** The process of identifying specific, measurable, achievable, relevant, and time-bound (SMART) objectives.
- **Grounding techniques:** Strategies used to bring attention to the present moment and reduce feelings of anxiety or distress.
- **Guided meditation:** A meditation practice led by an instructor or through audio, providing direction and focus.
- **Healing:** The process of recovering from physical, emotional, or psychological pain or trauma.

- **Healthy boundaries:** Rules that establish how one wishes to be treated in relationships to preserve respect and safety.
- **Healthy coping mechanisms:** Positive strategies for dealing with stress or emotional discomfort.
- **Healthy habits:** Positive behaviors that contribute to overall physical and mental well-being.
- **Historical trauma:** Cumulative emotional and psychological wounds experienced by a group over time due to significant events or oppression.
- **Inner child:** The representation of one's childhood self that holds memories, emotions, and experiences.
- **Inner wounds:** Emotional injuries or traumas from past experiences that affect present behavior and feelings.
- **Interpersonal relationships:** Connections or interactions between individuals that can have a significant impact on emotional health.
- **Journaling:** The practice of writing about one's thoughts, feelings, and experiences for self-reflection and healing.
- **Life satisfaction surveys:** Tools used to assess an individual's overall contentment with life and personal circumstances.
- **Limiting beliefs:** Negative thoughts that constrain one's potential and hinder personal growth.
- **Meditation:** A practice of focusing the mind to achieve mental clarity, relaxation, and a heightened state of awareness.
- **Mental health improvement:** Efforts made to improve psychological well-being and emotional stability.
- **Mind-body connection:** The relationship between a person's thoughts, feelings, and physical health.

- **Mindfulness:** The practice of being fully present and engaged in the current moment without judgment.
- **Mindfulness practices:** Techniques and exercises used to develop mindfulness, such as meditation and deep breathing.
- **Mindful breathing:** A mindful technique that involves concentrating on one's breath to improve relaxation and awareness.
- **Mood tracking:** Monitoring emotional states over time to recognize emotional patterns and triggers.
- **Negative self-beliefs:** Ingrained thoughts that create a poor self-image and self-worth.
- **Negative self-talk:** Internal dialogues that reinforce negative beliefs about oneself, leading to decreased self-esteem.
- **Overdependence:** Relying excessively on others for emotional support or decision-making, which causes unhealthy dynamics.
- **Parental relationships:** The connections and dynamics between individuals and their parents or guardians shaping emotional development.
- **Pattern recognition:** The ability to identify recurring behaviors or themes in one's life and relationships.
- **Personal boundaries:** Individual limits regarding emotional and physical space in relationships.
- **Personal goals:** Specific aspirations or objectives a person aims to achieve for personal development.
- **Personal growth:** The ongoing process of self-improvement and development in various life aspects.

- **Personal integrity:** Adhering to moral and ethical principles that define an individual's character and decisions.
- **Personal reflection:** The practice of introspection to assess one's thoughts, feelings, and behaviors for greater self-awareness.
- **Physical abuse:** Intentional harm inflicted on an individual through physical means.
- **Physical activity:** Any movement of the body that requires energy and contributes to physical health.
- **Physical self-care:** Activities aimed at caring for one's physical health and well-being.
- **Positive affirmations:** Constructive statements that promote a positive self-image and encourage personal growth.
- **Positive self-talk:** Internal dialogue that nurtures confidence, self-worth, and optimism.
- **Professional guidance:** Support and advice provided by trained professionals in mental health or personal development.
- **Reflection exercises:** Activities that encourage personal introspection and learning from life experiences.
- **Resilience:** The ability to adapt and bounce back from adversity, stress, or challenges.
- **Relationship dynamics:** The patterns of interaction, behavior, and communication between individuals in a relationship.
- **Reparenting:** The process of providing oneself with the care and guidance that may have been lacking in childhood.

- **Self-acceptance:** Embracing oneself fully, including strengths and weaknesses, and recognizing inherent worth.
- **Self-awareness:** The conscious knowledge of one's thoughts, feelings, and behaviors, which leads to better decision-making.
- **Self-compassion:** Being kind and understanding toward oneself in instances of suffering or perceived inadequacy.
- **Self-confidence:** A belief in one's abilities and judgment that strengthens self-assuredness.
- **Self-criticism:** The act of judging oneself harshly, often leading to negative feelings and self-doubt.
- **Self-discovery:** The process of exploring and understanding one's identity, values, and beliefs.
- **Self-doubt:** Uncertainty about one's abilities or self-worth, which may hinder personal growth.
- **Self-esteem:** One's overall sense of self-worth or personal value.
- **Self-exploration:** Using introspection to uncover feelings, thoughts, and motivations.
- **Self-identity:** The conception of oneself shaped by personal experiences, beliefs, and social contexts.
- **Self-love:** An appreciation for oneself that nurtures one's well-being and personal happiness.
- **Self-reflection:** The process of introspecting and evaluating one's thoughts, feelings, and behaviors.
- **Self-sabotage:** The act of undermining one's own goals and well-being through negative thoughts or behaviors.
- **Self-worth:** The intrinsic value one assigns to oneself, independent of external achievements or validation.

- **Sleep hygiene:** Practices and habits that improve quality sleep and overall well-being.
- **SMART goals:** Objectives that are Specific, Measurable, Achievable, Relevant, and Time-bound.
- **Social support:** The emotional, informational, or practical assistance received from others.
- **Support groups:** Gatherings of individuals sharing a common experience or challenge and providing mutual support.
- **Tension:** Mental or physical strain resulting from stress and leading to discomfort.
- **Therapeutic approaches/strategies/techniques:** Methods employed in therapy to promote healing and personal development.
- **Trauma:** An emotional response to a distressing event that can have lasting effects on an individual's mental health.
- **Trauma recovery:** The process of healing and growth following traumatic experiences.
- **Trauma-informed care:** An approach to understanding, recognizing, and responding to the effects of trauma on individuals.
- **Triggers:** Events or stimuli that provoke intense emotional reactions based on past experiences.
- **Unresolved issues:** Emotional conflicts or experiences that have not been adequately addressed or processed.
- **Vulnerabilities:** Areas of emotional sensitivity that can lead to feelings of hurt or insecurity.
- **Vulnerability in relationships:** The willingness to expose emotional risk and share personal feelings with others to foster closeness.

- **Visualization exercises/ techniques:** Mental practices that involve imagining positive scenarios or outcomes to improve emotional and mental well-being.
- **Yoga:** A practice that combines physical postures, breathing techniques, and meditation to promote holistic health and well-being.

REFERENCES

Ackerman, C. E. (2018, February 12). *Cognitive restructuring techniques for reframing thoughts*. Positive Psychology. https://positivepsychology.com/cbt-cognitive-restructuring-cognitive-distortions/

Attachment styles & CBT. (n.d.). My CBT. https://mycognitivebehavioraltherapy.com/attachment-styles-cbt

Benefits of mindfulness. (2024, August 30). HelpGuide.org. https://www.helpguide.org/mental-health/stress/benefits-of-mindfulness

Campbell, L. (2023, April 26). *Why personal boundaries are important and how to set them*. Psych Central. https://psychcentral.com/relationships/what-are-personal-boundaries-how-do-i-get-some

Cascio, C. N., O'Donnell, M. B., Tinney, F. J., Lieberman, M. D., Taylor, S. E., Strecher, V. J., & Falk, E. B. (2015). Self-affirmation activates brain systems associated with self-related processing and reward and is reinforced by future orientation. *Social Cognitive and Affective Neuroscience, 11*(4), 621–629. https://doi.org/10.1093/scan/nsv136

CBT and negative thought patterns. (n.d.). Your Journey Through. https://www.yourjourneythrough.com/blog/cbt-and-negative-thought-patterns

Celebrating progress: Recognizing achievements. (2024). BookBaker. https://www.bookbaker.com/ar/v/The-Path-to-Personal-Growth-A-Comprehensive-Guide-to-Self-Improvement-Celebrating-Progress-Recognizing-Achievements/8a3901e8-7059-444d-babb-e65bbe4d5218/31

Celebrating progress: Recognizing achievements in mental health. (2024, February 13). Positive Reset Eatontown. https://positivereseteatontown.com/celebrating-progress-recognizing-achievements-in-mental-health/

Celestine, N. (2021, June 2). *12 most reliable mental health assessment tools*. PositivePsychology.com. https://positivepsychology.com/assessment-tools/

Center for Substance Abuse Treatment. (2014). Understanding the impact of trauma. In *Trauma-Informed Care in Behavioral Health Services*. Substance Abuse and Mental Health Services Administration. https://www.ncbi.nlm.nih.gov/books/NBK207191/

Centers for Disease Control and Prevention. (2024, May 16). *About adverse childhood experiences*. U.S. Centers for Disease Control and Prevention. https://www.cdc.gov/aces/about/index.html

Chavan, K. P. (2023, November 4). *10 exercises to heal your inner child and why you need to heal yourself*. Medium. https://medium.com/@drketaki.oms/10-exercises-to-heal-your-inner-child-and-why-you-need-to-heal-yourself-d9bae1a1ec6a

Children's ABA therapy: Celebrating achievements in autism. (2024, January 18). Double Care ABA. https://doublecareaba.com/childrens-aba-therapy-celebrating-achievements-in-autism/

Clarke, M. (2019, April). *Transformative community: Culture of change*. Community Works, Inc. https://www.cworksindy.com/cultureofchange

Cohen, J. R., Menon, S. V., Shorey, R. C., Le, V. D., & Temple, J. R. (2017). The distal consequences of physical and emotional neglect in emerging adults: A person-centered, multi-wave, longitudinal study. *Child Abuse & Neglect, 63*, 151–161. https://doi.org/10.1016/j.chiabu.2016.11.030

Cooks-Campbell, A. (2022, March 15). *How inner child work enables healing and playful discovery*. BetterUp. https://www.betterup.com/blog/inner-child-work

Copley, L. (2024, March 29). *Reparenting: Seeking healing for your inner child*. PositivePsychology.com. https://positivepsychology.com/reparenting/

Cortez, P. A., da Silva Veiga, H. M., Stelko-Pereira, A. C., Lessa, J. P. A., Martins, J. Z., Fernandes, S. C. S., Priolo-Filho, S. R., Queluz, F. N. F. R., Trombini-Frick, L., & Peres, R. S. (2023). Brief assessment of adaptive and maladaptive coping strategies during pandemic. *Trends in Psychology*. https://doi.org/10.1007/s43076-023-00274-y

Doll, K. (2019, March 23). *23 resilience building activities & exercises for adults*. PositivePsychology.com. https://positivepsychology.com/resilience-activities-exercises/

Downey, C., & Crummy, A. (2021). The impact of childhood trauma on children's wellbeing and adult behavior. *European Journal of Trauma & Dissociation*, 6(1). https://doi.org/10.1016/j.ejtd.2021.100237

Dye, H. L. (2019). Is emotional abuse as harmful as physical and/or sexual abuse? *Journal of Child & Adolescent Trauma*, *13*, 399–407. https://doi.org/10.1007/s40653-019-00292-y

Ferguson, S. (2022, October 27). *Approval-seeking behaviors: signs, causes, and how to heal*. PsychCentral. https://psychcentral.com/blog/what-drives-our-need-for-approval

Ferris, E. (2023, November 7). *Self-Compassion: The key to healing and building resilience*. The Breath Effect. https://www.thebreatheffect.com/self-compassion-the-key-to-healing-and-building-resilience/

Garey, J. (2023, October 30). *How to change negative thinking patterns*. Child Mind Institute. https://childmind.org/article/how-to-change-negative-thinking-patterns/

Gillespie-Lopes, C. (n.d.). *Mindfulness and guided imagery: Scripts to help children cope with anxiety and stress*. Eluna Network. https://elunanetwork.org/resources/guided-imagery-use-these-scripts-to-help-children-cope-with-anxiety-and-str

Gillis, K. (2022, February 19). *10 ways childhood trauma can manifest in adult relationships*. Psychology Today. https://www.psychologytoday.com/us/blog/invisible-bruises/202202/10-ways-childhood-trauma-can-manifest-in-adult-relationships

Glowiak, M. (2024, January 23). *What is self-care and why is it important for you?* Southern New Hampshire University. https://www.snhu.edu/about-us/newsroom/health/what-is-self-care

Gowmon, V. (2021, April 16). *Take your childhood adversity seriously and you take a stand for your inner child*. Vince Gowmon. https://www.vincegowmon.com/take-your-childhood-adversity-seriously-and-you-take-a-stand-for-your-inner-child/

Grinspoon, P. (2022, May 4). *How to recognize and tame your cognitive distortions*. Harvard Health. https://www.health.harvard.edu/blog/how-to-recognize-and-tame-your-cognitive-distortions-202205042738

Grist, A. (2020, May 14). *Reparenting: responding to your inner child*. Amy Grist. https://amygrist.com/reparenting-responding-to-your-inner-child/

Gupta, S. (2023, May 25). *The importance of self-reflection: How looking inward can improve your mental health*. Verywell Mind. https://www.verywellmind.com/self-reflection-importance-benefits-and-strategies-7500858

Hines, K. L. (2022, July 5). *18 best journal apps for therapy and mental wellness*. Kristi Hines. https://kristihines.com/best-journal-apps-for-therapy/

Hood, J. (2020, February 3). *The benefits and importance of a support system*. Highland Springs. https://highlandspringsclinic.org/the-benefits-and-importance-of-a-support-system/

How and why to practice self-care. (2022, March 14). Mental Health First Aid. https://www.mentalhealthfirstaid.org/2022/03/how-and-why-to-practice-self-care/

How to manage and reduce stress. (2022). Mental Health Foundation. https://www.mentalhealth.org.uk/explore-mental-health/publications/how-manage-and-reduce-stress

Hundley, M. (2022, October 27). *The power of communication in A relationship*. Healing Collective Therapy. https://healingcollectivetherapy.com/resources/power-of-communication-in-a-relationship

Journaling to increase self-awareness. (n.d.). Prosper. https://prosper.liverpool.ac.uk/postdoc-resources/reflect/journaling-to-increase-self-awareness/

Kamila & Tim. (n.d.). *How our wounded inner child affect our lives?* Liberation Journey. https://liberationjourney.com/wounded-inner-child/

Kane, A. (n.d.). *The path to healing requires commitment*. A Lust for Life. https://www.alustforlife.com/tools/the-path-to-healing-requires-commitment

Kolyane, P. (n.d.). *The blueprint for lifelong personal growth: Unlocking success at every stage of your life*. Motivation and Success

Strategies | GetMotivation.
https://www.getmotivation.com/motivationblog/2024/02/bluepri
nt-for-lifelong-personal-growth/

Koosis, L. A. (2024, September 30). *The science of affirmations: The brain's response to positive thinking*. MentalHealth.com.
https://www.mentalhealth.com/tools/science-of-affirmations

Kuhfuß, M., Maldei, T., Hetmanek, A., & Baumann, N. (2021). Somatic experiencing–effectiveness and key factors of a body-oriented trauma therapy: a scoping literature review. *European Journal of Psychotraumatology, 12*(1).
https://doi.org/10.1080/20008198.2021.1929023

Lebow, H. I. (2021, June 10). *How Childhood Trauma May Affect Adult Relationships*. Psych Central. https://psychcentral.com/blog/how-childhood-trauma-affects-adult-relationships

Lew, B., Chistopolskaya, K., Osman, A., Huen, J. M. Y., Talib, M. A., & Leung, A. N. M. (2020). Meaning in life as a protective factor against suicidal tendencies in Chinese University students. *BMC Psychiatry, 20*. https://doi.org/10.1186/s12888-020-02485-4

Lynch, S. M., Keasler, A. L., Reaves, R. C., & Bukowski, L. T. (2007). The story of my strength: An exploration of resilience in the narratives of trauma survivors early in recovery. *Journal of Aggression, Maltreatment, & Trauma, 14*, 75–97.
https://www.researchgate.net/publication/232442735_The_Story_
of_My_Strength_An_Exploration_of_Resilience_in_the_Narratives_
of_Trauma_Survivors_Early_in_Recovery

MacWilliam, B. (2023, March 5). *Healing the inner child: Using inner child work to overcome codependency*. Codependency Recovery Council. https://codependencyrecovery.org/2023/03/05/healing-the-inner-child-using-inner-child-work-to-overcome-codependency/

Marie, V. (2023, September 2). *Why self-care is so important to heal from trauma*. Vanessa Marie Life Coach.
https://www.vanessamarielifecoach.com/post/self-care-heal-from-trauma

Martinez, S. (2023, May 9). *18 mental health activities for coping with stress, anxiety, depression, and more*. Ellie Mental Health.
https://elliementalhealth.com/18-mental-health-activities-for-coping-with-stress-anxiety-depression-and-more/

Matheka, W. (2023, March 4). *Reconnecting with your inner child*. Wendy Matheka. https://www.wendymatheka.com/post/reconnecting-with-your-inner-child

Mayo Clinic. (2023a, December 14). *Meditation: A simple, fast way to reduce stress*. Mayo Clinic. https://www.mayoclinic.org/tests-procedures/meditation/in-depth/meditation/art-20045858

Mayo Clinic. (2023b, December 23). *Resilience: Build skills to endure hardship*. Mayo Clinic. https://www.mayoclinic.org/tests-procedures/resilience-training/in-depth/resilience/art-20046311

Miles, J. R. (n.d.). *The science of visualization: What Jim Carrey can teach you*. John R. Miles. https://johnrmiles.com/the-science-of-visualization-jim-carrey/

Mindfulness exercises. (2022, October 11). Mayo Clinic. https://www.mayoclinic.org/healthy-lifestyle/consumer-health/in-depth/mindfulness-exercises/art-20046356

Mindfulness STOP skill. (n.d.). Cognitive Behavioral Therapy Los Angeles. https://cogbtherapy.com/mindfulness-meditation-blog/mindfulness-stop-skill

Mindset Makeover. (2023, July 12). *Embracing vulnerability: The path to personal growth and a healed heart*. Medium. https://mbbshrabdullah.medium.com/embracing-vulnerability-the-path-to-personal-growth-and-a-healed-heart-4d4cc2ec581f

Mohatt, N. V., Thompson, A. B., Thai, N. D., & Tebes, J. K. (2014). Historical trauma as public narrative: A conceptual review of how history impacts present-day health. *Social Science & Medicine, 106*, 128–136. https://doi.org/10.1016/j.socscimed.2014.01.043

Monfared, J. (2023). *Childhood trauma and its effect on adulthood*. Concept Palo Alto University. https://concept.paloaltou.edu/resources/business-of-practice-blog/childhood-trauma

Mortazavizadeh, Z., Göllner, L., & Forstmeier, S. (2022). Emotional competence, attachment, and parenting styles in children and parents. *Psicologia: Reflexão E Crítica, 35*. https://doi.org/10.1186/s41155-022-00208-0

Mosunic, C. (n.d.-a). *10 mindfulness questions to help you check in with yourself*. Calm. https://www.calm.com/blog/check-in-with-yourself

Mosunic, C. (n.d.-b). *Visualization meditation: 8 exercises to add to your practice*. Calm. https://www.calm.com/blog/visualization-meditation

Moyal, K. A. (2023, August 6). *5 steps to healing old relationship wounds that keep resurfacing*. Therapy and Co. https://therapyandcohouston.com/steps-to-healing-old-relationship-wounds/

Nash, J. (2018, January 5). *How to set healthy boundaries & build positive relationships*. Positive Psychology. https://positivepsychology.com/great-self-care-setting-healthy-boundaries/

Nash, J. (2022, October 16). *Expressive arts therapy: 15 creative activities and techniques*. PositivePsychology.com. https://positivepsychology.com/expressive-arts-therapy/

National Institutes of Health. (2021, June). *Mindfulness for your health*. NIH News in Health. https://newsinhealth.nih.gov/2021/06/mindfulness-your-health

National Institutes of Health. (2022). *Emotional wellness toolkit*. National Institutes of Health (NIH). https://www.nih.gov/health-information/emotional-wellness-toolkit

Neediness, boundaries, & reparenting your inner child: "Good inside" by Dr. Becky Kennedy. (2023, May 25). David Tian. https://davidtianphd.com/masculine-psychology-podcast/neediness-boundaries-reparenting-your-inner-child-good-inside/

Neff, K. (2024). *What is self-compassion?* Self-Compassion. https://self-compassion.org/what-is-self-compassion/

Patel, Y. (2023, July 12). *Embracing personal growth: A journey of self-discovery and fulfillment*. Medium. https://yash-patel.medium.com/embracing-personal-growth-a-journey-of-self-discovery-and-fulfillment-ec16953b5fd4

Peri, C. (2021, June 7). *What lack of sleep does to your mind*. WebMD. https://www.webmd.com/sleep-disorders/features/emotions-cognitive

Pikorn, I. (2019, August 30). *How to connect with and heal your inner child*. Insight Timer Blog. https://insighttimer.com/blog/inner-child-meaning-noticing-healing-freeing/

Ramirez de Arellano, M. A., Lyman, D. R., Jobe-Shields, L., George, P., Dougherty, R. H., Daniels, A. S., Ghose, S. S., Huang, L., & Delphin-Rittmon, M. E. (2014). Trauma-focused cognitive-behavioral therapy for children and adolescents: Assessing the evidence. *Psychiatric Services, 65*(5), 591–602. https://doi.org/10.1176/appi.ps.201300255

Reblin, M., & Uchino, B. N. (2018). Social and emotional support and its implication for health. *Current Opinion in Psychiatry, 21*(2), 201–205. https://doi.org/10.1097/yco.0b013e3282f3ad89

Relationships and communication. (2014). Better Health. https://www.betterhealth.vic.gov.au/health/healthyliving/relationships-and-communication

Resolutions vs. intentions: A new approach to self-improvement. (2024, January 11). Blue Umbrella. https://www.blueumbrellapsychiatry.com/resolutions-vs-intentions-a-new-approach-to-self-improvement

Rob, G. (2024, August 13). *The importance of self-reflection for personal growth*. Medium. https://medium.com/@golamrob/the-importance-of-self-reflection-for-personal-growth-16ecded5c97b

Robinson, L., & Smith, M. (2024, August 21). *Stress management: Techniques & strategies to deal with stress*. HelpGuide.org. https://www.helpguide.org/mental-health/stress/stress-management

Robson, D. (2021, January 13). *Why self-compassion—not self-esteem—leads to success*. BBC. https://www.bbc.com/worklife/article/20210111-why-self-compassion-not-self-esteem-leads-to-success

Rohde-Brown, J. (2023). Shadow and society: The forgotten child in collective contexts. *Journal of Jungian Scholarly Studies, 18*. https://jungianjournal.ca/index.php/jjss/article/download/224/137

Salzgeber, N. (2017, June 20). *Why high achievers choose self-compassion over self-criticism*. NJlifehacks. https://www.njlifehacks.com/self-compassion-versus-self-criticism/

Self-kindness: Definition, benefits, and techniques. (2023, July 6). Modern Recovery Services. https://modernrecoveryservices.com/wellness/coping/skills/emotional/self-kindness/

Selhub, E. (2022, September 18). *Nutritional psychiatry: Your brain on food*. Harvard Health Publishing. https://www.health.harvard.edu/blog/nutritional-psychiatry-your-brain-on-food-201511168626

Shukla, A., Choudhari, S. G., Gaidhane, A. M., & Quazi Syed, Z. (2022). Role of art therapy in the promotion of mental health: A critical review. *Cureus, 14*(8). https://doi.org/10.7759/cureus.28026

Sonu, S., Mann, K., Potter, J., Rush, P., & Stillerman, A. (2024). Toward integration of trauma, resilience, and equity theory and practice: A narrative review and call for consilience. *The Permanente Journal, 28*(1), 1-18. https://doi.org/10.7812/tpp/23.105

Spelman, B. (2023, March 10). *Healing inner child wounds: The essential guide to reparenting*. Private Therapy Clinic. https://theprivatetherapyclinic.co.uk/blog/healing-inner-child-wounds/

Stanborough, R. J. (2023, June 5). *How to change negative thinking with cognitive restructuring*. Healthline. https://www.healthline.com/health/cognitive-restructuring

Sutton, J. (2016, July 21). *Active listening: The art of empathetic conversation*. Positive Psychology. https://positivepsychology.com/active-listening/

Sutton, J. (2022, October 8). *Inner child healing: 35 practical tools for growing beyond your past*. PositivePsychology.com. https://positivepsychology.com/inner-child-healing/

Sutton, J. (2024, January 17). *SMART goals, HARD goals, PACT, or OKRs: What works?* PositivePsychology.com. https://positivepsychology.com/smart-goals/

Tartakovsky, M. (2022, May 2). *8 daily habits to boost mental health – and signs it may be time to get support*. Healthline. https://www.healthline.com/health/mental-health/habits-to-improve-mental-health

10 daily habits to improve your mental health. (2023, November 8). The Haven Detox. https://arkansasrecovery.com/10-daily-habits-to-improve-your-mental-health/

10 somatic interventions explained. (n.d.). Integrative Psychotherapy & Trauma Treatment. https://integrativepsych.co/new-blog/somatic-therapy-explained-methods

The importance of celebrating milestones in recovery. (2024, July 30). The
Wave Columbia. https://www.thewavecolumbia.com/blog/the-
importance-of-celebrating-milestones-in-recovery

Thompson, R. J., Mata, J., Jaeggi, S. M., Buschkuehl, M., Jonides, J., &
Gotlib, I. H. (2010). Maladaptive coping, adaptive coping, and
depressive symptoms: Variations across age and depressive state.
Behaviour Research and Therapy, *48*(6), 459–466.
https://doi.org/10.1016/j.brat.2010.01.007

Tiret, H. (2023, February 13). *Active listening and empathy for human
connection*. Michigan State University.
https://www.canr.msu.edu/news/active-listening-and-empathy-
for-human-connection

Umberson, D., & Karas Montez, J. (2020). Social relationships and health:
A flashpoint for health policy. *Journal of Health and Social
Behavior*, *51*(1), 54–66.
https://doi.org/10.1177/0022146510383501

Understanding emotional triggers and building healthy relationships.
(2024, June 16). Sunshine City Counseling.
https://www.sunshinecitycounseling.com/blog/emotional-
triggers-and-relationship-issues-in-therapy

Watson, S. (2023, November 20). *Serotonin: The natural mood booster*.
Harvard Health Publishing. https://www.health.harvard.edu/mind-
and-mood/serotonin-the-natural-mood-booster

Webster, E. M. (2022). The impact of adverse childhood experiences on
health and development in young children. *Global Pediatric
Health*, *9*(9). https://doi.org/10.1177/2333794x221078708

Wedge, M. (2021, April 14). *Reflections on Alice Miller*. Psychology Today.
https://www.psychologytoday.com/za/blog/suffer-the-
children/202104/reflections-alice-miller

West, M. (2022, April 20). *Can exercise help stress, anxiety, and
depression?* MedicalNewsToday.
https://www.medicalnewstoday.com/articles/how-does-exercise-
reduce-stress

Wilson, C. (2021, April 22). *What is self-sabotage? How to help stop the
vicious cycle*. PositivePsychology.com.
https://positivepsychology.com/self-sabotage/

Wooll, M. (2022, June 28). *Own your personal development: self-improvement goals that motivate*. BetterUp. https://www.betterup.com/blog/goals-for-self-improvement

Wright, K. W. (2023, November 2). *Building self-awareness: How to use journaling to know yourself better*. Day One | Your Journal for Life. https://dayoneapp.com/blog/self-awareness/

Wright, S. A. (2021, November 8). *How to identify and overcome trauma triggers*. Psych Central. https://psychcentral.com/health/trauma-triggers

Yoon, Y. (2023, December 23). *Building authentic connections: Embracing vulnerability*. Psychology Today. https://www.psychologytoday.com/us/blog/on-second-thought/202312/building-authentic-connections-embracing-vulnerability

Zeinali, A., Sharifi, H., Enayati, M., Asgari, P., & Pasha, G. (2011). The mediational pathway among parenting styles, attachment styles and self-regulation with addiction susceptibility of adolescents. *Journal of Research in Medical Sciences, 16*(9), 1105–1121. https://www.ncbi.nlm.nih.gov/pmc/articles/PMC3430035/

Zhuo, M. (2024). "I feel my inner child out": Zine-making as a data collection tool in narrative inquiry. *Research Methods in Applied Linguistics, 3*(3). https://doi.org/10.1016/j.rmal.2024.100131

www.ingramcontent.com/pod-product-compliance
Lightning Source LLC
Chambersburg PA
CBHW052313220526
45472CB00001B/96